Shobana R. Vinay

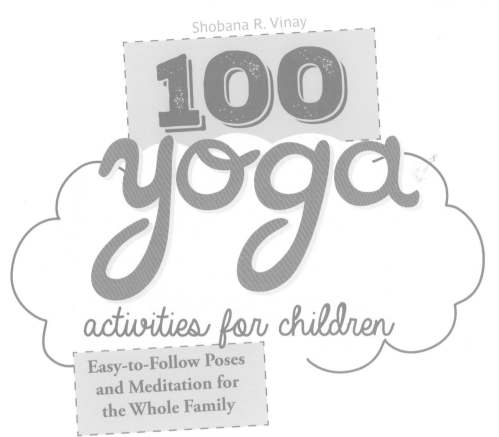

100 yoga
activities for children

Easy-to-Follow Poses and Meditation for the Whole Family

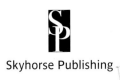

Skyhorse Publishing

Table of Contents

Meditation and Relaxation

relaxation

meditation

breathing

flexibility

mudras or gestures

Yoga

Standing poses

trikonasana
50. Difficult – *Ugrasana*

Introduction

Yoga is an ancient Indian practice that was introduced to western culture during the late nineteenth century. Through controlled breathing and various simple or complex postures, yoga improves flexibility, releases mental and physical tensions, and boosts energy. Thousands of years ago, the yogis who developed *asanas* (poses) were living in close contact with nature, from which they drew most of the posture's names: swan's grace pose, tree pose . . .

It is generally accepted that children are master imitators; they will gladly join you in a yoga practice.

Starting yoga early provides a practice of lifelong discipline and an array of health benefits. Physically, yoga develops self-awareness through flexibility, strength, and coordination between body and mind.

Yoga also develops concentration, appeasement, and relaxation.

Children are so flexible and have such a good sense of balance that they actually can get into poses much more easily than adults. Most of them are receptive to yoga; they might just need a little encouragement at first!

In their everyday lives, children today are often not very close to nature. They experience different types of stress caused by the demands of numerous activities. They evolve in a world fraught with competition, social media, new technologies, and a sense of urgency. Many sensorial stimuli are constantly bombarding their brains, which consequently process a heavy load of information without getting enough rest.

Even very early on in life, learning to breathe and to center our attention through meditation are excellent ways to empty our mind while at the same time expanding our mental capacity.

It is also generally accepted that children don't have a very long attention span. Paired with *mudras*—simple, entertaining gestures that resemble mini-yoga poses for hands—meditation improves concentration. They also activate pressure points on hands or fingers to regulate the body's five elements, which in turn helps children to rapidly find calm and assurance. Each mudra has specific results and healing powers.

In schools where meditation is taught, teachers have noticed a quantifiable improvement in their students' work and behavior.

How to organize the sessions

To prepare the body, start with a warm-up exercise. Then quickly transition into a breathing exercise (with or without meditation or mudra). Continue with a sequence of several poses.

If the child asks, you can add yogic games and end by a complete body relaxation (p. 14).

The benefits of the poses can be divided into two main categories: mental and emotional needs and motor skills. Prepare your program by choosing poses whose specificity addresses the needs or wishes of your child.

Mental benefits

To release stress:
All the meditation poses: crocodile, happy baby, reclining hero, inverted triangle.

To improve concentration and balance:
Tree, mountain, warrior III, kite, inverted triangle, supported headstand, tree.

To stimulate memorization and dissipate fear or vertigo:
All head-down poses: supported headstand, half-supported headstand, downward-facing dog, difficult, brain yoga.

Physical benefits

All the beginner postures are accessible to younger children. The intermediate and advanced postures can be practiced once they reach five years of age. For the advanced poses (half-supported headstand, camel, etc.), it is imperative that a parent be present.

Poses can be practiced in sequence. Offer to practice variations one after the other. From a forward, backward, or sideways bend, the child can go into pendulum; from a forward bend, into triangle, arc, cobra, tortoise, moon arc, and plow.

Regarding twisting poses, there is fish—sitting or lying variations—and inverted triangle.

For hip flexibility:
One-legged king pigeon, extended side angle, garland, sleeping Vishnu (side-reclining leg stretch), warrior I, II, and III.

For leg, ankle, and foot strength:
Chair, star, warrior I, II, and III, tree, kite, triangle, ferocious.

For arm, shoulder, wrist, and hand strength:
Upward plank (or toboggan), plank, tabletop, staff, wheel, upward-facing dog.

For the digestive system and abs:
Diamond, bow, child, locust, half-boat.

Fun and playful postures:
Cat (meowing), cow (mooing), lion (roaring), cobra (hissing), bow (foot by the ear, like a telephone), frog, upward plank (or toboggan), plank (ball running down the back), kite (pretend flight), chair (Kangaroo jumps), tiger, upward-facing dog, table.

To easily find each activity, please refer to the alphabetical index on the back flap of this volume.

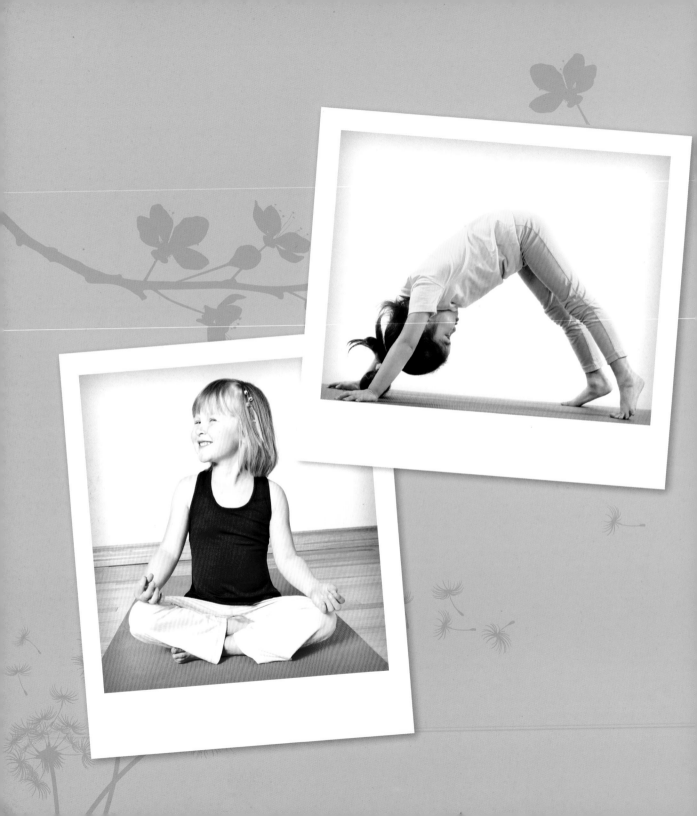

Meditation and relaxation

In order to meditate and be relaxed, one has to concentrate and breathe properly. The first sessions detailed within this book deal with meditation, which implies concentration—too abstract a notion for young children. To help them concentrate and reach relaxation, we will therefore use touch meditation that calls on their sense of touch.

Through meditation, your child also develops a breathing practice. In an effort to maintain their attention, the posture explanations are rather playful and refer to animals or nature to speak to the younger group.

The flexibility exercises prepare the body for yoga postures, with simple poses working on the neck, arm, legs, and knee muscles or joints.

Because they link concentration and breathing, *mudras* ("gesture" in Sanskrit) look like hand yoga. They balance the body, which is composed—just like the universe—of five elements. Each finger is associated with one part of the body: the thumb corresponds to fire; the index to air; the middle finder to space; the ring finger to earth; and the pinkie to water. In the same way, by stimulating the reflexive zones, each zone of the palm and of each finger interacts with a part or organ of the body.

Summary

Relaxation - activities 1 to 5

Meditation - activities 6 to 11

Breathing - activities 12 to 16

Flexibility - activities 17 to 21

Mudras - activities 22 to 32

1 THE HEAD

This exercise aims to relax the muscles in the face and brings a feeling of relaxation and appeasement by releasing accumulated tensions. The session also promotes feeling through touch: the child visualizes the part of the body on which your finger travels.

1. Tell your child their head is like a mountain. This trip starts at the top of the mountain to end at the bottom of the valley.

2. Put your fingers on the top of the head, i.e. the top of the mountain.

3. Go down the forehead, traveling along its entire surface and explaining to the child that it is a mountain lake.

4. Go onto both brows that you describe as two pine forests.

5. Outline the eyes while explaining that they are two bumps that have worked hard since the morning.

6. Do not forget the two ears, the two cliffs that have listened a great deal and now need some rest.

7. Go back on the cheeks and describe them as mountain slopes that need to relax to receive more kisses.

8. Then the nose, a peak that functions during our whole life and deserves to relax.

9. Then go down towards the lips and the mouth. End the trip on the chin, the last bump before the abrupt valley. The mountain—the face—is now relaxed.

Activities 1 to 5 aim to reestablish contact with one's body by simple gestures that will prove to be very beneficial. These sessions can take place any time, preferably in a calm setting. The child is lying on their back, on a yoga mat, or a bed, eyes closed and arms alongside the body. The parent is close to the child, speaking calmly, with fingers slowly going from one part of the child's body to the other, using images to describe it. The child has to concentrate on each part of their body while listening to the story.

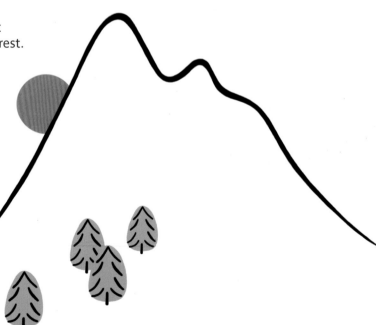

2 FROM NECK TO HIP

In this session, touch targets the arms and the torso (respiratory and digestive organs). The upper part of the body is particularly active in a growing child and will greatly benefit from relaxation.

1. Tell your child to imagine their neck is a bridge that links the mountain to the plain. Put your fingers on the abrupt valley of the chin, and slowly move downward to reach the large bridge. This is essential, for it links the mountain (the head) with the plain (the body) by allowing communication from the head to the rest of the body.

2. Turn to reach the shoulders, which have been instrumental in moving the arms all day. Continue onto the arms, these two long cliffs above an unknown sea, coming out of the continent and stretching all the way to the tip of the fingers.

3. Slowly move back up the arms to the shoulders and the large plain of the torso: moving, living, throbbing plain under which the heart of the earth—and of the body—is pulsating.

4. Feel the breathing, the heart beating while slowly traveling onto the torso with your fingers. The trip continues toward the rest of the plain that, just like the surface of the planet Earth, moves up and down, experiencing tremors with every breath. And under this plain, there is a factory that brings life to the whole body.

5. Travel onto your child's belly while explaining that the food is digested to fuel the body.

6. Move left or right to reach one of the hips, each of which links half of the body weight to the leg.

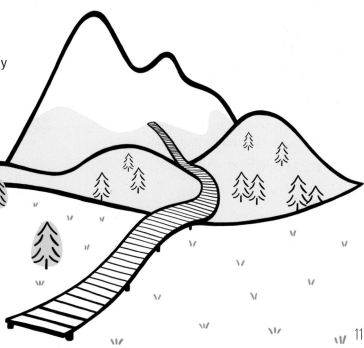

11

3. FROM HIP TO TOES

The bottom part of the body supports the child's weight and contributes to its mobility. Its muscles are quite taxed.

1. Travel onto the stomach plain in order to reach the hip plain that has supported the upper body all day. Tell your child the hips have to take a break and relax.

2. Now, move down the legs—these two rivers that have helped your child walk, run, and jump all day. Don't they also deserve to rest?

3. Midway, you meet the whirlpool of the knee that has worked hard moving and bending. Your finger turns and turns around the kneecap to relax it.

4. When the knee is well-rested, move on to the second half of the river.

5. The lower part of the knee is a waterfall with rapids forming on the tibias. They also are tense after an active day.

6. At the end of the river, you find yourself in the small lake of the ankle, which can now relax after having been the prisoner of a shoe all day.

7. Now, you are ascending the two rocky peaks that hold the body up during the day, which can now relax and rest.

8. Behind the rocky peaks, visit the arches. Move back and forth on each toe to end up on the biggest one, which is also the highest.

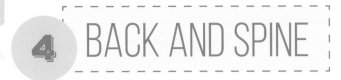

4 BACK AND SPINE

The back of the body is essentially used to sit or stand, while the spine determines our flexibility. Both the back and the spine are much in demand at school or while playing. Concentrating on them as the child lies face down provides muscle relaxation and tension release.

1. For this session, your child is prone on their stomach. Start with the mountain of the head, and slide down on the neck that has held up the head all day. Explain that the head is now at rest. Then discover the vast desert plain of the back, with its central axis made of aligned rocks, the vertebras of the spine.

2. Softly apply your finger on each one, feeling the spine. The spine allows the child to stand, remain seated, and is now taking a well-deserved rest.

3. At the base of the spine, continue your trip by ascending the mountains of the buttocks.

4. Each of these mountains gives way to two rivers that you carefully travel down to reach the river of the thigh.

5. Once your reach the back of the knee, circle there for a while so as to relax this often tense part.

6. Continue the trip down the leg, and turn your attention to the heel. It has carried the weight of the whole body and now deserves to relax.

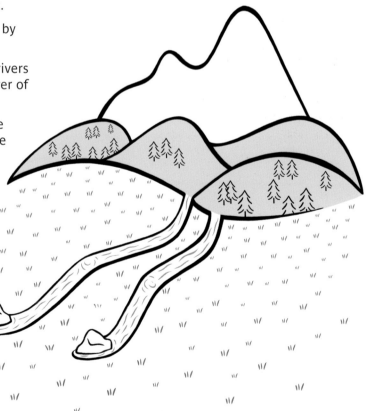

5 THE WHOLE BODY *Savasana*

This exercise is a shorter version of the four previous ones. Its aim is to perfect the gestures required for each body meditation session. Touch relaxation brings a feeling of well-being, calm, and concentration to the child. It diminishes mental and muscular stress and improves the quality of self-awareness and self-confidence.

1. Start with your child's head. With your finger, move around the face, touching the eyes, the nose, the mouth, and the ears. Explain the function of each and remind the child that they have to rest. The face has looked, listened, and talked all day and now needs to relax.

2. The trip continues onto the torso, the shoulders, the arms, the hands, and the fingers. All these parts have been moving and now deserve some rest. All day, the upper body has been breathing, moving, and digesting. Time to rest and relax!

3. Move up the arms, torso, and stomach, ending up on the hips. Describe the vital functions of the heart. Then, from the hips, move down the thighs, the knees, the feet, and the toes. The lower half of the body is essentially dedicated to movement; its muscles have been taxed and now need to relax. Explain to your child the effort their body expends every day and insist on the importance of resting.

4. Turn the child on their stomach and let your finger travel along the back. Underline the essential function of the spine, then that of the buttocks, the legs, and finally the feet. They all participate in the child's movements. The back and buttocks—which we often forget about—also have to relax: they

allow us to remain upright. The trip ends with the essential role of the feet and heels that support the weight of the whole body.

5. This meditative voyage has ended. The child is now full of energy after a well-deserved rest.

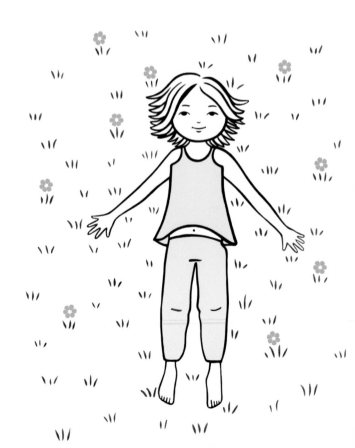

6 LEGS-UP-THE-WALL 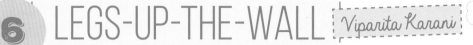 *Viparita Karani* *beginner*

This pose brings rest and well-being to the child by inverting blood circulation in the legs and increasing blood flow to the top part of the body.

To get into these meditation poses (activities 6 to 11), the child must be totally confident. If necessary, use a mat or a cover. Do the exercise with the child. Support their spine in a straight position, and the lower part of the body arched so they can sit for a long enough time. Also ask the child to sit against a wall so their back is perfectly straight. Have the child relax their shoulders, neck, and jaw, and breathe calmly through the nose while concentrating on breathing and on the air that comes in and out of the nostrils. Concentration will be improved by keeping the eyes shut.

Young children should hold the pose for five minutes (tell them a story or put on some music). The older ones can hold the pose for fifteen minutes.

1. Lie on your back.

2. Lift your feet up, and extend your legs against a wall. If necessary, place a cushion in the small of your back and under your buttocks. Keep your eyes closed.

3. The body should be at a right angle to the floor and the wall.

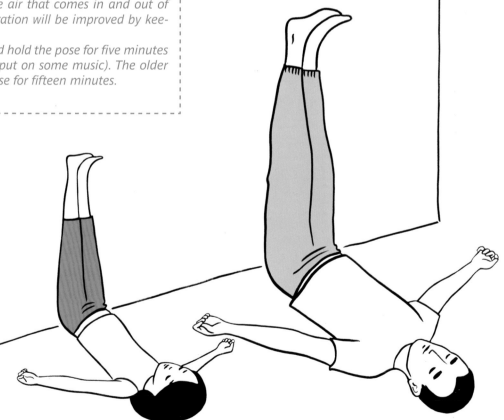

15

7 POND Tadagasana

This pose helps the child relax and rest by loosening the muscles.

1. Lie on your back, legs slightly apart.
2. Bend your legs so your feet are flat on the floor.

3. Bring your arms up above your head. Hold this relaxing position for at least five minutes, breathing normally.

4. Come back to the original position by placing your legs and arms on the floor.

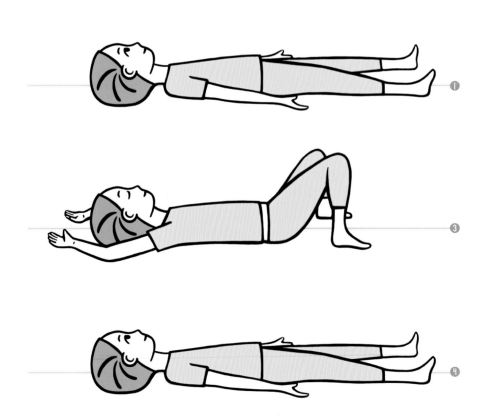

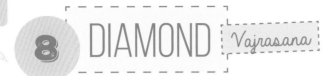

8 DIAMOND *Vajrasana*

This pose helps the child relax and find peace. It fosters blood circulation and digestion.

1. Sit on your heels.

2. Your spine is straight, the small of your back nicely arched.

3. Relax your shoulders, neck, and jaw.

4. Put your palms on your thighs.

5. Breathe calmly through your nose, concentrating on your breathing. Close your eyes to hone your concentration.

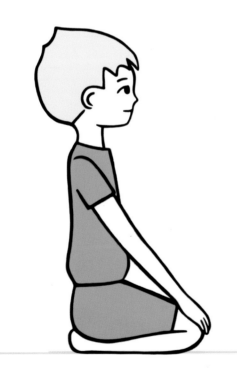
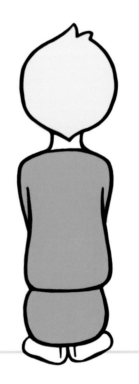

9 EASY *Sukhasana*

This pose helps the child relax and find peace. It is recommended before meditation and mudra practice.

1. Sit crossed-legged on the floor. Your spine should be straight, and the small of your back nicely arched.

2. Relax your shoulders, neck, and jaw. Breathe calmly through your nose.

3. Close your eyes to improve concentration.

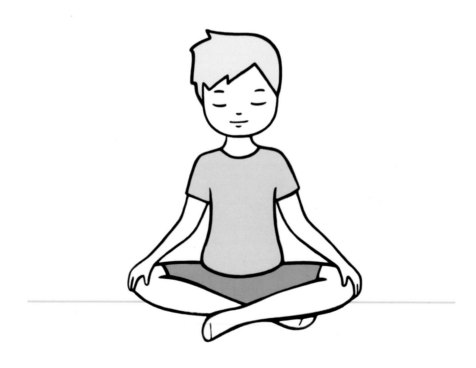

10 LOTUS AND HALF-LOTUS

Padmasana et ardha padmasana

This pose helps the child relax and find peace. It promotes blood circulation and digestion. It works the ankles and relaxes the hips.

1. Sit with your legs extended in front of you.

2. Using your hands, bring one foot onto the opposite thigh, as close to the hip as possible.

3. Repeat with the other foot. Start with the one that seems easier to you to avoid straining your muscles. It is usually easier to start with the right side.

4. If you're unable to perform this pose, choose the half-lotus: place your first foot as described, then simply place the other foot under the thigh.

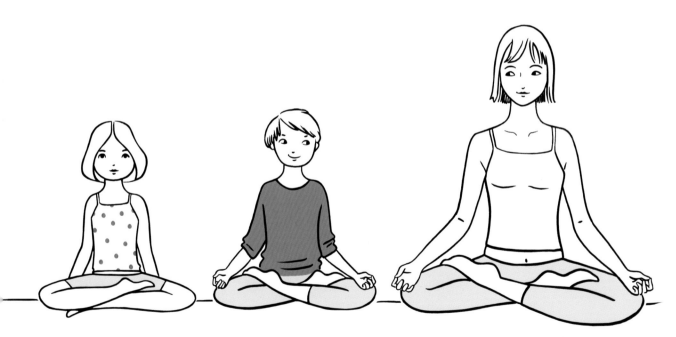

demi-lotus   lotus

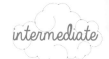

11 ACCOMPLISHED *Siddhasana*

This pose helps the child relax and find peace. It is recommended before meditation and mudra practice.

1. Sit with your legs extended in front of you

2. Using your hands, bring your right heel as close as possible to your pelvis.

3. Place your left foot on top of the right leg. Your two ankles need to be one on top of the other. Begin with either foot.

4. Keep your spine straight, the small of you back nicely arched. Relax your shoulders, neck, and jaw.

Breathe calmly through your nose, concentrating on your breathing. Close your eyes.

5. Do the chin-mudra: place your hands on your thighs, join your index fingers and your thumbs on each hand, and keep the three other fingers extended.

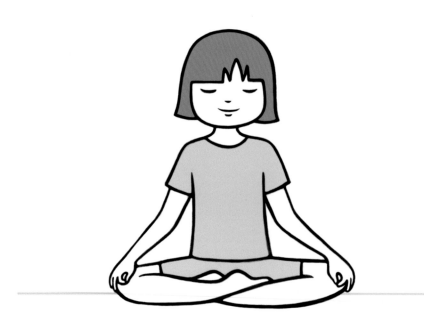

12 MOUNTAIN Tadasana

An imaginary walk in nature inspires this playful breathing pose. Breathing well brings life, and more importantly, a better quality of life.

1. For this exercise, you need to be sitting down. Four sitting positions are possible for this pose: easy (p.18), diamond (p.17), lotus (p.19), or half-lotus (p.19). Go a little further than what your body can do naturally, but never force too much. In order to succeed, you need to be calm and relaxed.

2. Envision yourself as a mountain. Extend one of your arms so the tips of your fingers form the peak. Use the index and middle fingers of your other hand to mime a little person who is about to climb up to the top of the mountain.

3. As the climber slowly goes from your shoulder up to the tips of your fingers, breathe slowly through your slightly open mouth.

4. Once on top of the mountain and taking in the view, the little person eventually has to come back down: walk your hand down as you are slowly breathing out by letting the air very slowly flow out of your mouth.

5. The hike is so enjoyable that the little person decides to climb up and down the mountain several times.

Practice these breathing exercises (activities 12 to 16) with your child. The playful poses teach the younger children to breathe properly and to control their breath. Breathing is the basis of several athletic and artistic activities, such as singing or running. In our every day life, breathing enables us to control our emotions. Breathing is necessary to our yoga practice because each component of a yoga pose corresponds to an inhale or an exhale. Breathing sessions can be practiced anywhere, anytime.

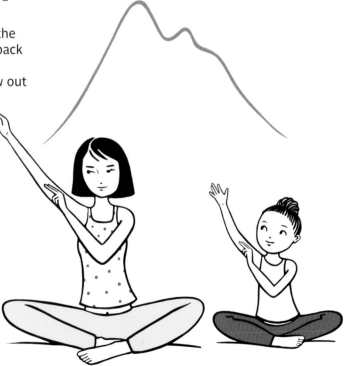

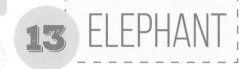

13 ELEPHANT

This type of breathing exercise is composed of an inhaling and an exhaling phase. The image of an elephant that takes in water to spray itself provides a visual metaphor that helps children understand breathing cycles. This comprehension is essential to the exercise.

1. Stand up with your feet together.

2. You are an elephant that is using its trunk to suck water from a lake and then blow it out. Put one hand on top of the other and bring your arms down, palms towards you, to represent the trunk.

3. Bend down as far as you can.

4. Without modifying your hand position, slowly come back up while breathing gently and making the sound of water being sucked up: the elephant is drawing water from the lake with its trunk.

5. Once you are standing straight up with your arms above your head, slowly bend down again, gently exhaling while making the sound of water being continuously expelled: the elephant is spraying water with its trunk

6. Repeat the exercise several times, very calmly.

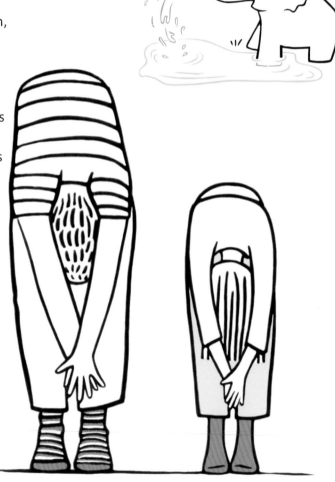

14 PEACOCK *Mayarusana*

Sitting in a relaxed position allows your child to experience the regulatory impact of breathing on our nervous system and our blood circulation. Physiologically, breathing is really essential.

1. Sit or stand with your feet together and extend your arms out to the sides so they are parallel to the ground. Four sitting positions are possible for this pose: easy (p.18), diamond (p.17), lotus (p. 19), or half-lotus (p.19).

2. You are a peacock. Like this beautiful bird, you display your feathers. Slowly bring your extended arms up while inhaling with your lips half-closed.

3. Gently bring your hands together above your head.

4. Eventually, the peacock closes its tail. Without rushing, make a semi-circle down while exhaling very gently.

5. You can repeat this exercise several times, calmly.

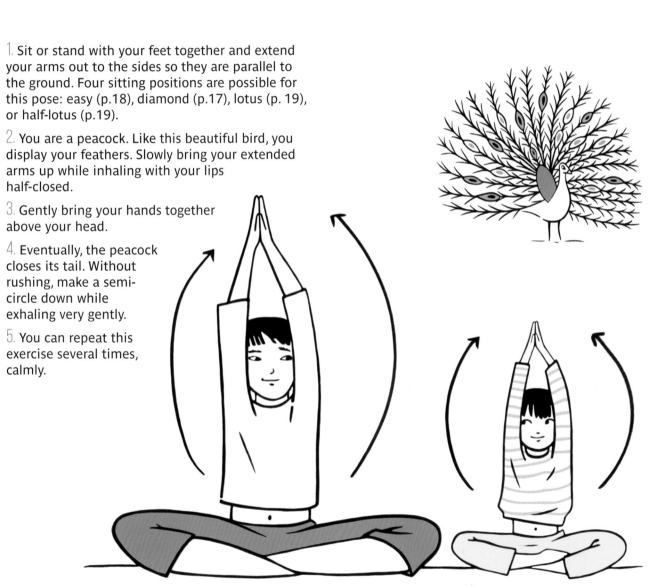

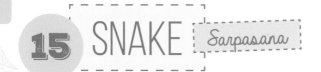

15 SNAKE *Sarpasana*

Breathing and emotions interact: feelings affect breathing and vice-versa.

1. Sit on your heels, with your legs bent.

2. Bring your palms together above your head.

3. Go as far down as you can, and place your hands away from you.

4. You are going to envision yourself as a snake and hiss just like one. Place your tongue against your palate. Slowly raise your head while inhaling, letting the air flow between your tongue and your palate.

5. When your arms are vertical, bring your head back down as you exhale while letting air out and hissing continually. You become a snake hissing to protect itself.

6. You can repeat this exercise several times, calmly.

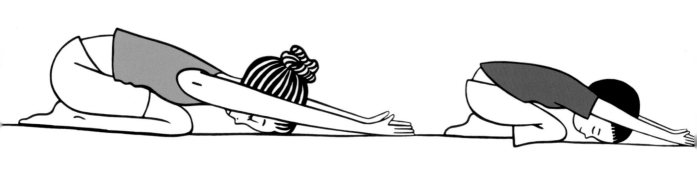

16 BUTTERFLY *Badha Konasana*

Modern life does not pay much attention to the role of breathing. Breathing enables us to control our emotions and recover our calm when we're stressed. Using the image of a butterfly inhaling and exhaling the nectar of a flower as a fun visual aid, children can experience the value of the breath by utilizing this pose.

1. Visualize yourself as a butterfly who's just landed on a flower and is about to take in some nectar. Sit down, with your back straight and your legs extended in front of you.

2. Slightly bend your knees and place the soles of your feet against each other. Wrap your hands around your toes.

3. You are now a butterfly. Bend your torso forward, until you can touch your feet with your forehead, if you can without forcing too much.

4. Come back up slowly while inhaling.

5. Once your back is straight, slowly exhale through your mouth. The butterfly is slowly breathing out some of the nectar.

6. You can repeat this exercise several times, calmly.

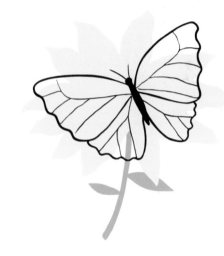

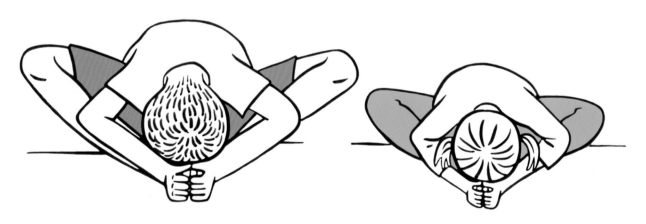

17 ARMS *Hasta sanchalan*

This pose strengthens and loosens the child's neck, arms, and shoulders.

1. Lie on your back, with your legs slightly apart. Extend your arms along your body and raise them up a few inches. Bring both arms up in a semi-circle so your hands are both above your head. Clasp your hands and turn your palms outward while stretching your whole body from head to toe. It is helpful to push the soles of your feet towards the floor. Come back to your initial position, with your arms alongside your body.

2. Extend your arms upward, bringing them above your head. Clasp your hands, then turn your palms outward while stretching your whole body from head to toe. Come back to your initial position, arms along the body.

3. Arms are extended, slightly off the floor along your body. Using a semi-circular side motion, bring your arms above your head and back down above your stomach, making several scissor movements. Come back to your initial position, arms along the body.

These flexibility exercises (activities 17 to 21) are perfect as an introduction into yoga. They also work on your child's flexibility, "oil" the articulations, and maintain their muscles. They should be practiced in a relaxed environment, without straining. You can use your imagination and add head movements (yes, no, perhaps, etc.) or shoulder swimming, etc.

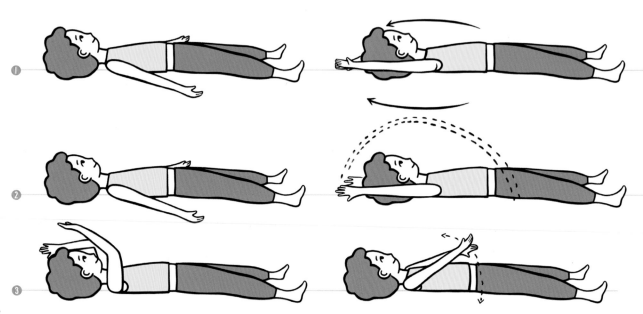

18. FEET · Padha sanchalan

This pose loosens the child's thighs, hips, legs, and ankle articulations.

1. Lie on your back. Bend your left leg while keeping your foot on the floor, so the base of your heel touches your left buttock. Bend the right leg while keeping your foot on the floor, so that the base of your heel touches your right buttock. Bend both arms and place them under your head. Stretch your whole body, from your head to the small of your back.

2. Extend both legs. Lift your left leg and make a circular movement with your foot, slowly and smoothly. Repeat three times. Switch legs.

3. With your arms extended on the floor, bring your arms up to align them with your shoulders, creating in a large T. Keeping your head on the floor, flip your left leg so your left foot touches your right hand. Come back to your initial position. Switch legs. Be gentle and fluid.

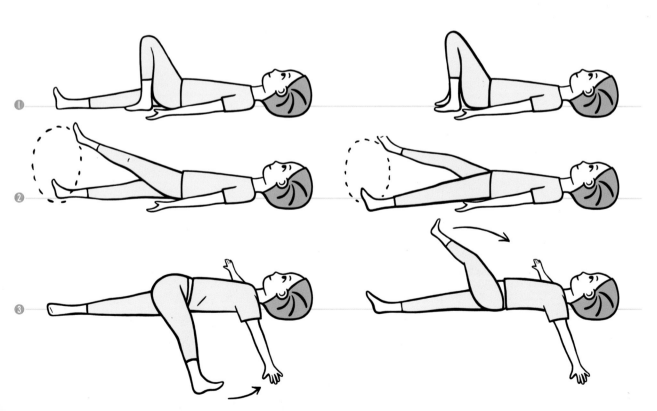

27

19 KNEES *Janu sanchalan*

This pose strengthens and loosens the child's spine, knees, and hip.

1. Lie on your back, crossing your arms under your head. Bend your left leg, and, keeping your foot on the floor, place it as close to your hip as you can. Foot anchored on the ground, bring your left knee as close to the right of your hip as possible. Come back to your original position. Keeping your right foot on the floor, bend your right leg and place your foot as close to your hip as possible. Foot firmly anchored on the floor, bring your right knee as much to the left of your hip as possible. Come back to your initial position.

2. Keeping your left foot on the floor, bend your left leg so your foot comes as close to your hip as possible. The left leg must be bent at a forty-five-degree angle toward the outside. Foot anchored on the floor, bring your left knee to the right as much as

you can. Come back to your initial position. Keeping your foot on the floor, bend your right leg and place it as close to your hip as possible. The left leg must be at a forty-five-degree angle toward the outside. Foot firmly anchored on the floor, bring your right knee as much to the left as possible. Come back to your initial position.

3. Bend your legs, put your soles together and bring your feet as close to your hips as possible. Bring your knees as much to the left as possible, while moving your head to the right. Come back to your initial position. Switch sides. Slowly repeat the movement three to five times.

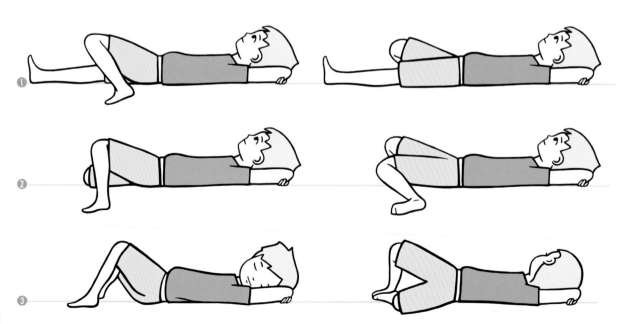

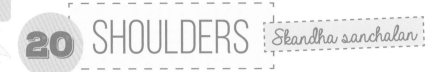

20 SHOULDERS Skandha sanchalan

This pose strengthens and loosens the child's shoulders.

1. Sit with your legs shaped like a diamond, i.e. legs bent and sitting on your heels. Both arms are relaxed.

2. Gently lift your shoulders trying to touch your ears. Bring them back down slowly. Repeat three to five times, gently.

3. Arms bent, place the tips of your fingers (not the thumbs) on your shoulders. Slowly rotate your elbows so they touch in front of you. Repeat three times in each direction.

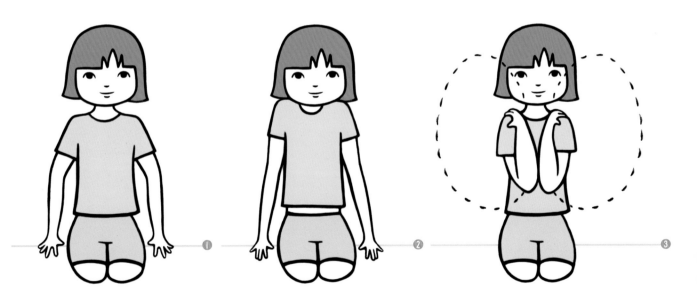

21 NECK *Kantha sanchalan*

This pose strengthens and loosens the child's neck.

1. Sit with your legs shaped like a diamond, i.e. legs bent and sitting on your heels. Gently tip your head forward so your chin touches your torso. Then gently tip your head backward so the back of your head touches the top of your back.

2. Turn your head to the right, then to the left. Gently tip your head to the left so your left ear touches the left shoulder. Then tip it to the right so the right ear touches the right shoulder. Repeat three to five times, gently and slowly.

3. Move your head successively: to the front so your chin touches your torso; to the left so your left ear touches your left shoulder; backwards so the back of your head touches the top of your back; to the right so your right ear touches your right shoulder. Switch sides. Repeat three to five times on both sides, slowly and gently.

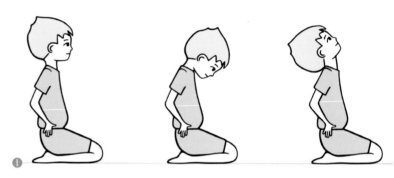

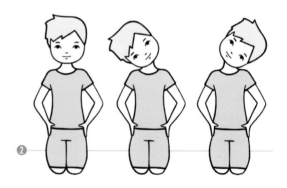

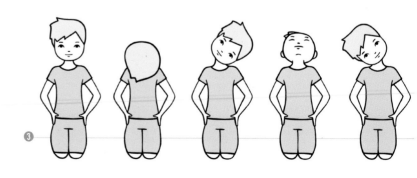

22 SALUTATION MUDRA Anjali-mudrâ beginner

This gesture reduces stress and mental anxiety. It is therefore used to appease the child's mind. It brings peace and love. Because all the fingers are involved, this mudra brings harmony to body and mind.

Mudras (activities 22 to 32) are hand and finger movements that can be practiced any time, anywhere. Nonetheless, it is recommended to practice them sitting, or in one of the following three yoga postures: easy (p.18), diamond (p.17), lotus or half-lotus (p.19).
Practice the exercises with your child: five to fifteen minute-sessions with the older children; a minimum of ten deep breathing cycles through the nose for the younger ones. Choose simple mudras for the youngest (2½ to 4½ years old) and don't expect them to replicate them perfectly.
Make sure your child is relaxed; the pressure applied on the fingers must stay light. Eyes must be shut or looking directly ahead, breathing free. The regular practice of the mudras will bring noticeable, immediate, or somewhat delayed health benefits.

1. Sit in the easy pose, with your legs crossed.

2. Join your two hands, palm against palm at the level of your heart.

3. Keep looking straight in front of you, keeping your back and shoulders straight.

4. The forearms are parallel to the floor.

5. Hands are away from the torso, not resting on it.

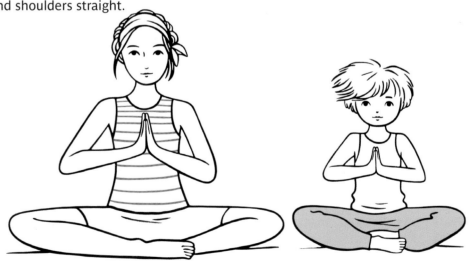

23 MEDITATION MUDRA

Dhyana-mudra

This gesture appeases your child and improves their concentration.

1. Sit comfortably in one of the four following poses: happy (p.18), diamond (p.17), lotus, or half-lotus (p.19).

2. Position your hands in dhyana-mudra, where your right hand is in your left hand, palms upwards, tips of the thumbs in contact, resting in the hallow of your legs.

3. Breathe normally, concentrating on your breathing.

Depending on your child's age, the exercise will last from three to fifteen minutes. Closing their eyes will enhance concentration.

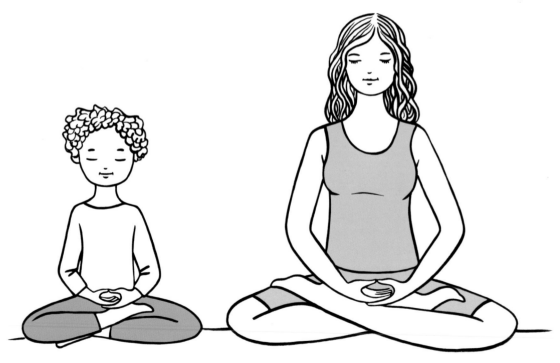

half-lotus

lotus

24 WISDOM MUDRA

Gnyana (Jnana) mudra

This gesture increases your child's concentration and helps memorization. Practiced regularly, it provides mental appeasement and calm.

1. Sit in easy pose, cross-legged.
2. Turn your palms upward.
3. Join the tips of your thumbs and index fingers.
4. Keep the other three fingers extended.

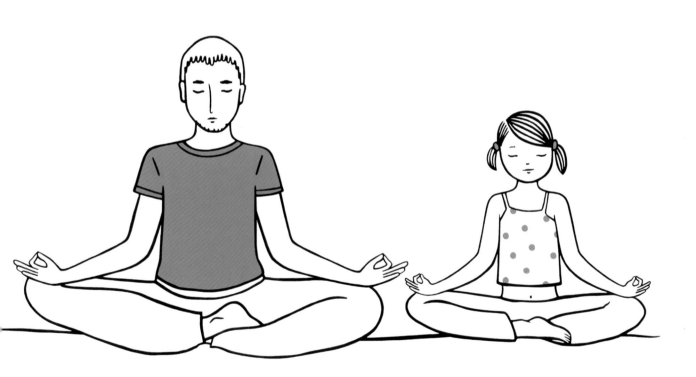

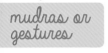

25 AIR MUDRA

Shunya-mudra

This gesture is recommended to calm your child's mind during meditation. It improves inner ear function by dissipating any associated pain. This posture helps to reduce fatigue and revitalize one's energy. It also increases patience.

1. Sit in easy pose, cross-legged.
2. Turn your palms upward.
3. Join the tips of your thumb and middle finger.
4. Keep the other three fingers extended.

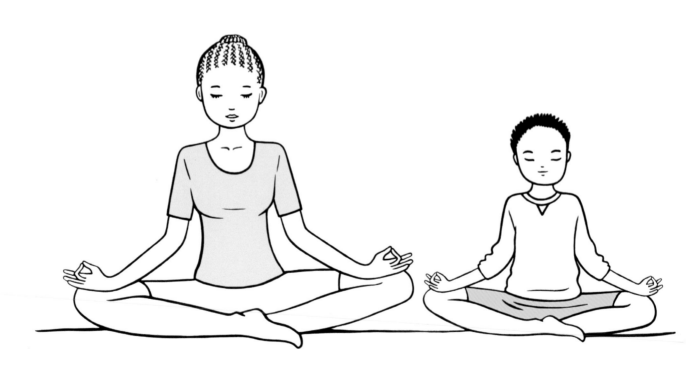

26 EARTH MUDRA Prithvi-mudra

This gesture helps balance the various elements in your child's body by strengthening it and alleviating fatigue. Its practice brings stability and self-confidence to the child.

1. Sit in easy pose, cross-legged.
2. Turn your palms upwards.
3. Join the tips of your thumbs and ring fingers.
4. Keep the other three fingers extended.

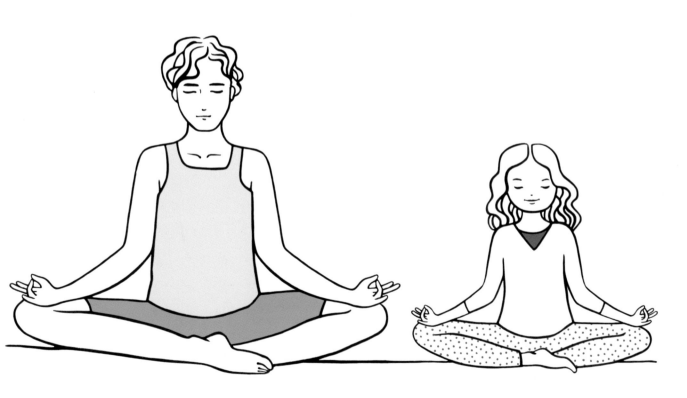

27 WATER MUDRA *Varuna-mudra*

This gesture improves the circulation of fluids in the body. It stabilizes the water level in the blood, while developing intuition and emotions. It also helps the child fight stomach flu and reduces muscle contractions.

1. Sit in easy pose, cross-legged.

2. Turn your palms upwards.

3. Join the tips of your thumbs and your pinkie fingers.

4. Keep the other three fingers extended.

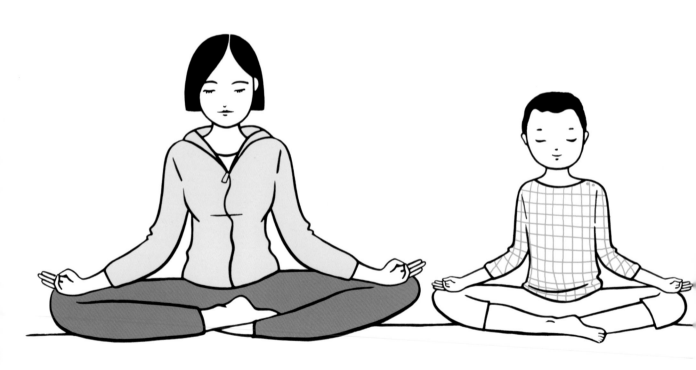

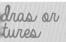
28 TURTLE IN THE SHELL MUDRA

Adhi-mudra

This gesture helps calm your child's nervous system. It facilitates lower abdomen breathing, while increasing vital lung capacity and oxygen flow in the throat and head.

1. Sit in easy pose, cross-legged.

2. Bring the tip of your thumbs to the base of your pinkies.

3. Bend the four other fingers of each hand, so as to hide your thumbs.

4. Join your loose fists, palms toward the sky, and then place your hands on your knees or thighs.

5. For this gesture to make more sense to your child, you can compare it to a snail hiding in its shell.

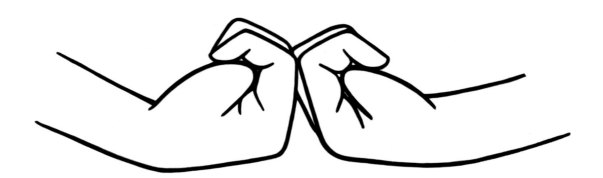

29 LIFE MUDRA *Prana-mudra*

This gesture helps cure a child's eye and sleeping problems. It shrinks blood vessel size and restores strength. When practiced regularly, it is an energy booster.

1. Sit in easy pose, cross-legged.

2. Bring the tips of your thumbs, your ring fingers, and your pinkie fingers together, while keeping the two other fingers of each hand extended.

3. Hands can now rest on the thighs or knees.

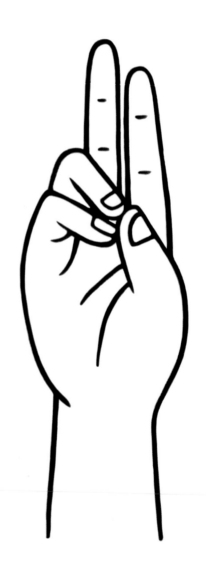

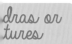
30 FIRE MUDRA *Surya-mudra*

This gesture restores physical strength, mobility, and vigilance; helps eliminate bad cholesterol; and benefits children who are sensitive to cold by keeping their body warm.

1. Sit in easy pose, cross-legged.

2. Turn the palms of your hands upwards. Bend the tips of your ring fingers so they touch the bases of your thumbs.

3. Softly bend the thumb over your ring fingers, keeping the other three fingers of both hands extended.

4. The hands can now rest on thighs or knees.

5. During practice, concentrate on the solar plexus.

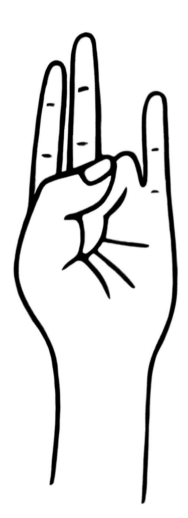

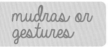

31 CONCENTRATION MUDRA

Akini-mudra

beginner

This mudra develops the child's cognitive ability by activating the connections between the right and left hemispheres of the brain. It improves the functioning of the brain and enhances memorization.

1. Sit in easy pose, cross-legged.

2. Join your fingertips, without having your palms touch.

3. The forearms can now rest on the thighs or the knees.

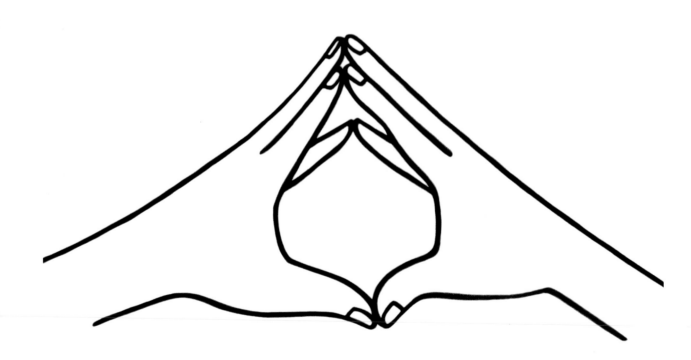

32 COURAGE MUDRA

Ahamkara-mudra

This gesture reinforces self-assurance and self-confidence. It helps dissipate fear and shyness. *Ahamkara* is a Sanskrit word used to describe egoism, vanity, or self-confidence.

1. Sit in easy pose, cross-legged.

2. Slightly bend both of your index fingers and position the tips of your thumbs on their second phalanxes.

3. Keep the three other fingers of each hand extended.

4. The hands can now rest on the thighs or the knees.

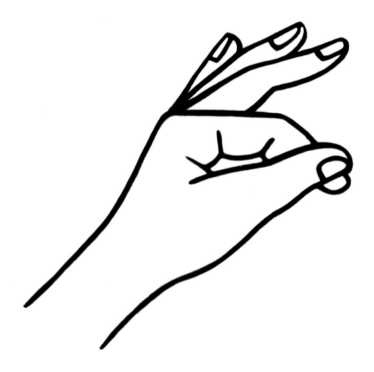

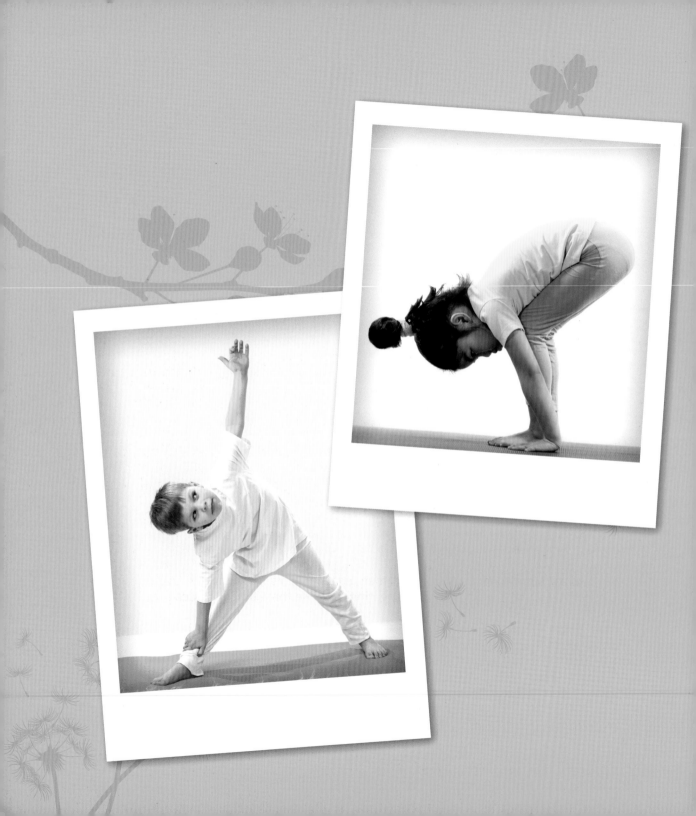

Yoga

This section provides a step-by-step description of the main yoga postures as well as more advanced poses—face, eyes, brain yoga—and yogic games. The standing, sitting, and lying postures are analyzed elsewhere in this volume. When you prepare your yoga session plan, combine the ideas from each section (see p. 5) to maximize your child's yogic experience and its subsequent benefits.

As you will see, the exercises in this book promote the health of the entire body. The standing poses develop concentration necessary to maintain balance. Standing poses that imply bending work on the muscles and joints. "Hand support" standing poses strengthen arms, wrists, and shoulders. By simple virtue of gravity, the "head down" standing poses increase the blood flow to the brain. The "legs apart" standing poses reinforce the leg muscles and open the pelvis. Eye yoga maintains eyeball muscles and improves vision. Face yoga resorts to funny faces to engage the numerous facial muscles. To further motivate your child to practice yoga, suggest yogic games that include making sounds, screaming, and breathing. These are generally quite a hit!

During the exercise, help your child improve their form, making sure the process is always gentle: the muscles and bones of this young body are still growing. Depending on age, interest, and flexibility, a session can last from fifteen to thirty minutes (a little longer if there is a real motivation), with a maximum of one hour. It is recommended that each pose be repeated three times. If the exercise calls for repeating the pose three times on each side, alternate sides!

Summary

33 MOUNTAIN *Tadasana*

A child's balance is imperfect; like the adult's, it oscillates. This pose enhances stability and corrects deviations of the vertebrae.

1. Stand up straight, feet 4" apart.

2. Keep the arms along the body, palms facing downward.

3. Slowly raise the arms a few inches.

4. Your fingers initiating the movement, bring your hands to a right angle with your arms.

5. Inhale and exhale deeply three times.

Because standing postures (activities 33 to 50) require no equipment and very little space, they can be practiced anytime, anywhere. They can be suggested to your child during a lengthy wait, possibly inviting other children and making it a group game. A "standing posture" can include a forward bending pose, a backward leaning pose (moon arc), a side leaning pose (angle), or a balance pose (tree or kite).

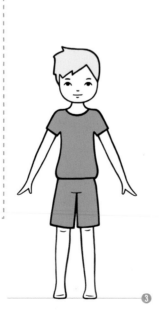
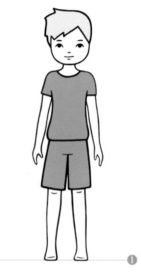
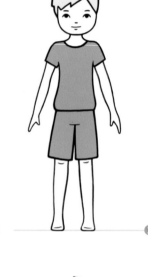
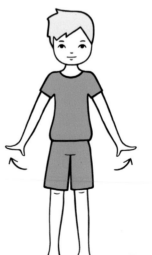
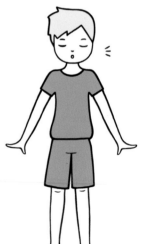

34 LORD OF THE DANCE *Natarajasana* *intermediate*

This pose develops your child's concentration, balance, and feet muscles as well as back and hip flexibility.

1. Stand with your back straight, shoulders slightly tilted backward, feet parallel.

2. Inhale deeply while raising your right arm above your head.

3. Bend your left leg backward and grab your left foot with your left hand.

4. Bend forward.

5. Come back to your initial position while exhaling.

6. Repeat three times. Switch sides.

Provide some help if your child experiences difficulty keeping the pose.

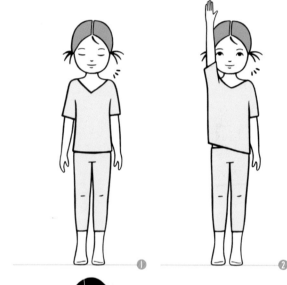

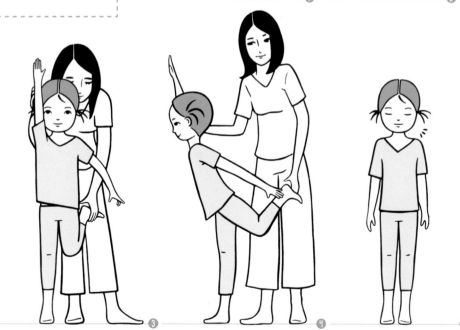

35 TREE *Vrkshasana*

This pose develops your child's concentration, balance, and feet muscles. It strengthens the legs and works on shoulder, hip, knee, and ankle flexibility. The arms' vertical movement opens the thorax and increases the blood flow to the heart.

1. Stand with your legs slightly apart.

2. One leg firmly anchored on the floor, start bending the other, heel turned inward.

3. Slowly bring the heel onto the knee of the other leg. If the child is able, you can help bringing the heel onto the thigh.

4. Bring your arms up, palms pointing to the ceiling.

5. While inhaling, join both hands above your head, arms extended. It is helpful to fix your gaze on a point straight ahead of you: ocular stability is essential to keep your balance.

6. Exhale while coming back to the original position. Switch sides. Repeat three times on each side.

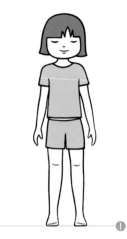

①

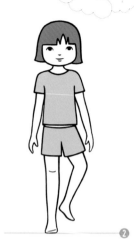

②

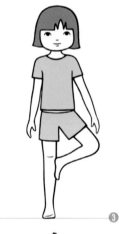

③

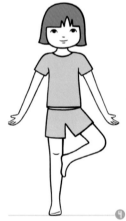

④

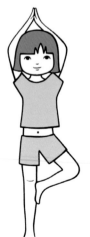

⑤

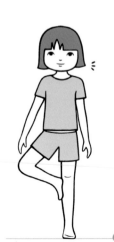

⑥

36 WARRIOR III Veerabadrasana III

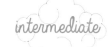

This pose improves the child's concentration and balance. It also reinforces the glutes, thighs, and abdominal muscles.

1. Standing feet together, breathe while bringing both arms over your head.

2. Exhale, while bending forward and raising one leg backwards so your arms, torso, and raised leg are aligned with the floor, if at all possible. Fix your gaze on one point on the floor or straight in front of you to keep your balance. Try to hold the pose a few seconds while breathing normally.

3. Inhale and come back to the original position, arms above your head.

4. Exhale while bringing your arms along your body.

5. Switch sides. Repeat two to three times on each side.

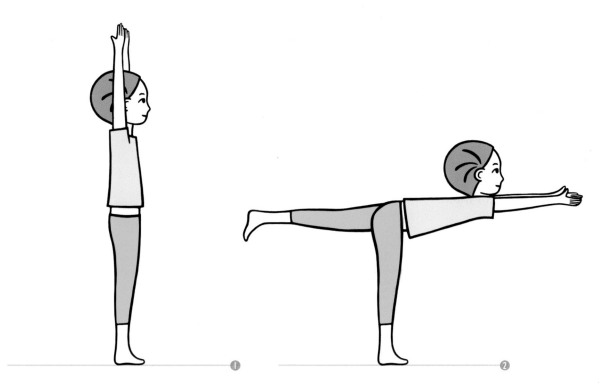

❶   ❷

37 KITE *Patangasana*

This pose is recommended to improve flexibility and stretch the child's torso, thighs, knees, and ankles. It also facilitates digestion.

1. Standing with your feet together, inhale while extending both arms out parallel to the floor.

2. As you exhale, bend forward while raising one leg up so your torso and raised leg are aligned with the floor, if possible. Look straight in front of you to keep your balance. Try to hold the pose for a few seconds while breathing normally.

3. Inhale as you go back to your initial position, feet together, arms still extended out. Exhale while bringing your arms down.

4. Switch sides. Repeat two to three times on each side.

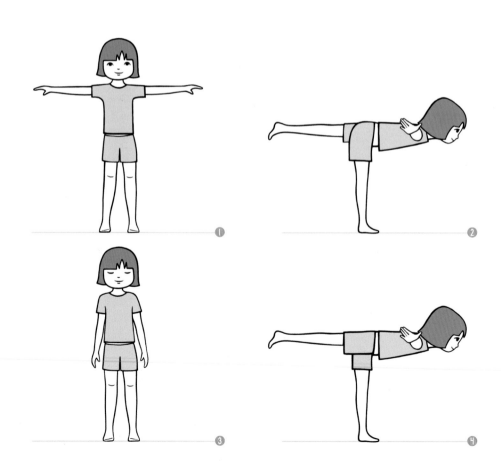

38 MOON ARC *Piraiasana*

This pose is recommended to improve the flexibility of your child's spine. Because it stretches the stomach muscles and the intestines, it also improves digestion.

1. Stand legs with your slightly apart.
2. As you inhale, slowly raise your arms.
3. Keep your arms extended.
4. Slightly bend backward.

5. Exhale while coming back to your original position.
6. Repeat three times.

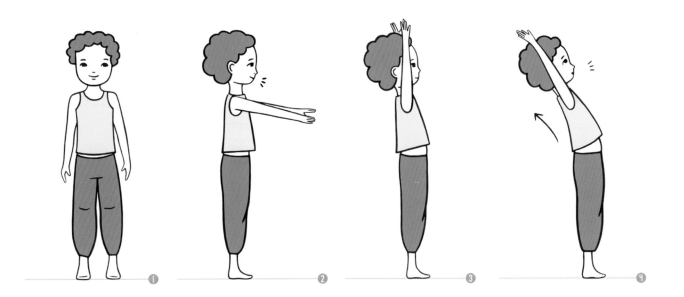

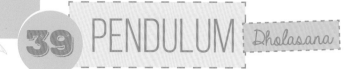

39 PENDULUM *Dholasana*

This pose improves the flexibility of your child's back. It develops stability and balance. It prepares for forward leaning poses, like river and giraffe.

1. Stand, legs slightly apart. Put both hands on the back of your head.

2. Bend forward so your head is at the level of your knees.

3. Using a pendulum movement, bring your head to your right knee then to your left knee.

4. Repeat this back and forth movement at least three times.

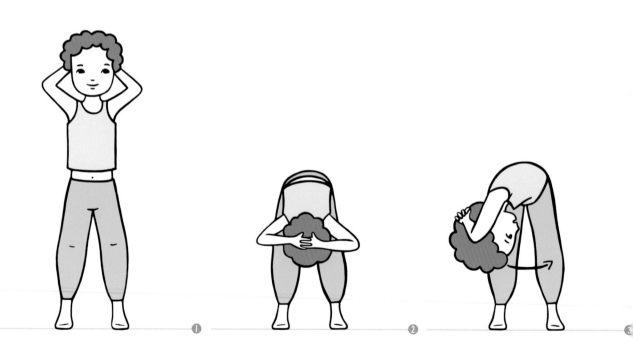

40 STANDING FORWARD BEND

Uttanasana

First and foremost, this pose benefits your child's back. It also engages the abdominal organs, and alleviates aerophagia and gastric difficulties.

1. Stand with your legs slightly apart.

2. As you inhale, bend forward and try to put your hands on your feet, keeping your legs straight. Go as far down as you can without straining your body.

3. Get back up while inhaling.

4. Repeat three times.

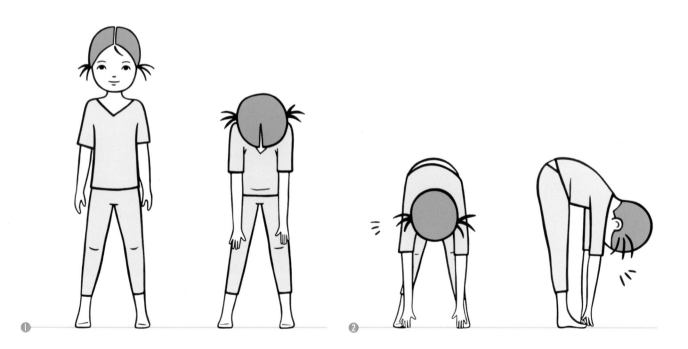

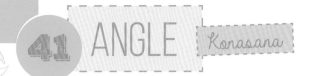

41 ANGLE *Konasana*

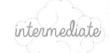

This pose represents the different phases of the moon. It stretches the back muscles and works the spine.

1. Stand with your legs apart. Inhale while bringing your arms up and join your hands above your head.

2. Stretch as much as you can to the right, while exhaling. Maintain the position for a few seconds, breathing normally.

3. Come back to the initial position.

4. Switch sides. Repeat three times on each side.

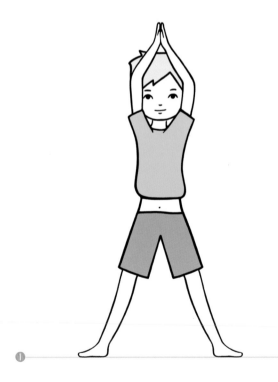

❶

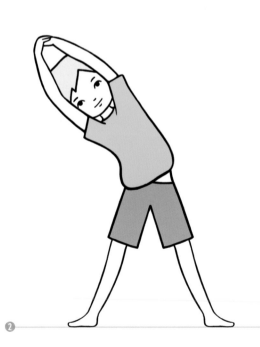

❷

42 CHAIR Utkatasana

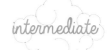

This pose stretches your child's spine while reinforcing their lower back, legs, thighs, and soles. It stimulates balance, the abdominal organs, the diaphragm, and the heart.

1. Stand back straight, feet together, arms extended in front of you. Inhale.

2. Bend your knees while exhaling and pretend you are sitting on a chair. Maintain this position for a few seconds.

3. Inhale as you come back to the initial position.

4. Repeat three times.

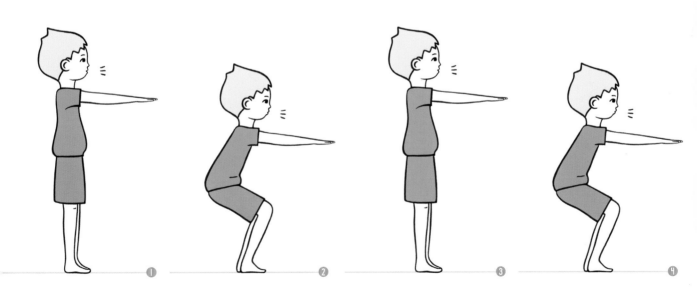

43 CRANE *Bakasana*

This pose develops your child's balance, coordination, and concentration. It works the arms, hands, shoulders, and abdominal muscles. It also provides an active back stretch.

1. Start in a standing position.

2. Bend forward looking down. Your arms are slightly bent, resting on an imaginary knee-high table.

3. Bend one of your legs back to assume the position of the crane.

4. Come back to your initial position. Switch sides and maintain the pose for a few moments.

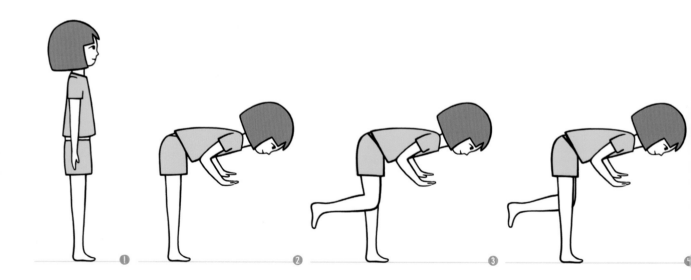

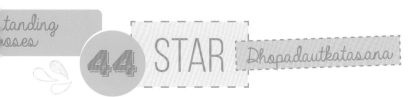

44 STAR *Dhopadautkatasana*

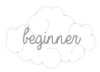

This standing pose, which helps keep the spine straight, develops your child's balance and concentration. It works the legs and improves blood circulation.

1. Stand, keeping your spine straight.

2. Inhale while bringing your legs apart and extending your arms horizontally, palms toward the floor.

3. Stay in the star position while exhaling and inhaling a few times.

4. On an exhale, come back to your initial position.

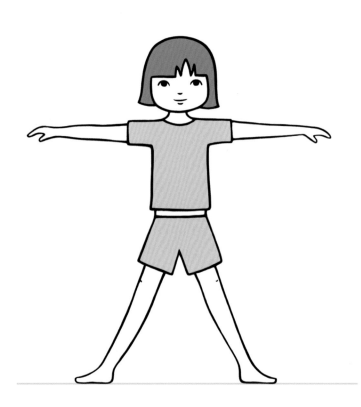

45 WARRIOR I Veerabadrasana I

This pose develops your child's thorax. It opens the hips; strengthens the legs, thighs, and knees; stretches and strengthens the chest, shoulders, neck, stomach. and groin. This pose also strengthens arm and back muscles. It improves endurance and strength, particularly in the legs and ankles.

1. Standing, bring your right leg forward and bend it. Your left leg is extended.

2. Your front foot is perpendicular to your back foot and remains flat.

3. Extend both your arms up. Slightly tilt your head back and look at your arms.

4. Keep the pose a few seconds while breathing slowly. Come back to your initial position.

5. Switch sides. Repeat three times, alternating sides.

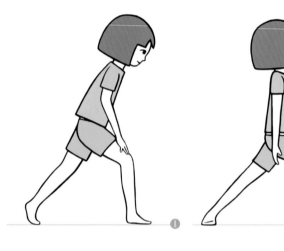

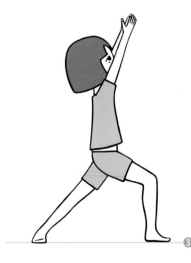

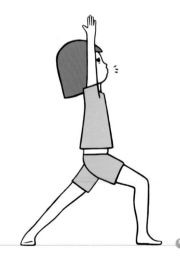

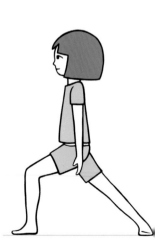

46 WARRIOR II

Veerabadrasana II

This pose develops your child's thorax. It opens the hips; strengthens the legs, thighs, and knees; stretches the chest, shoulders, neck, stomach, and groin. Additionally, the pose strengthens the shoulder, arm, and back muscles of the child and improves endurance and strength, particularly in the legs and ankles.

1. Standing, bring your right leg forward and bend it. Your left leg is extended.

2. Your front foot is perpendicular to your back foot, which remains flat.

3. Twist your torso without moving your head, still looking forward.

4. Extend your left arm forward and your right arm backward. Stay in that position for a few seconds while breathing slowly. Come back to your initial position.

5. Switch sides. Repeat three times, alternating sides.

Help your child if they experience difficulty with some of the movements.

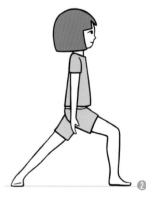

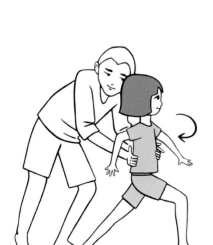

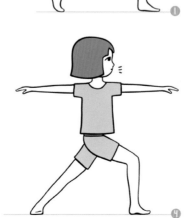

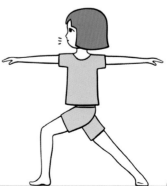

47 EXTENDED SIDE ANGLE

Utthita parsva konasana

This pose helps your child create space between their shoulders and stretch their pelvis. It stretches the lateral back muscles, brings flexibility to the spine and knees, and tones the thighs.

1. Stand up, legs wide apart. Inhale while raising both arms horizontally, palms facing downward.

2. Bend the right knee while twisting the foot outward.

3. Exhale while bending your right side laterally, positioning your right hand flat at the back of the right foot.

4. Extend your left arm over your head, touching your left ear. The body must be in a straight line from the left arm to the left foot. Keep the pose for a few seconds while breathing normally.

5. Come back to your original position and switch sides.

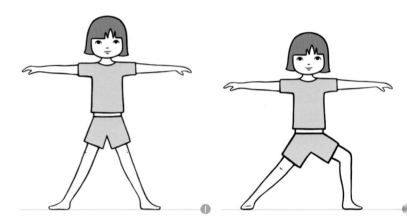

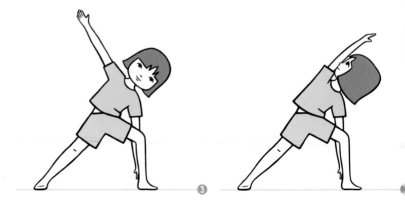

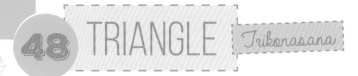

48 TRIANGLE *Trikonasana*

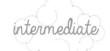
This pose loosens the child's vertebrae. The twisting motion massages the intestines and improves digestion.

1. Stand up, legs wide apart.

2. Extend your arms out shoulder height, palms facing downward.

3. Inhale deeply as you stretch your arms out horizontally.

4. and 5. Bend your torso to the right and position your right hand flat on your right foot as you exhale. Your left arm and hand are extended, your gaze as high as possible.

6. Come back to your original position and switch sides.

7. Repeat three times, alternating sides.

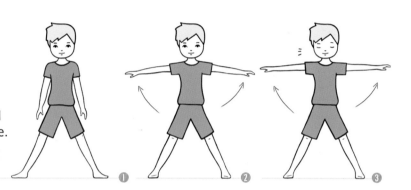

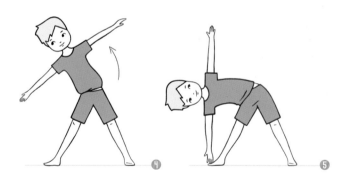

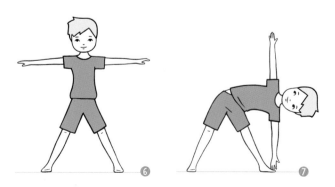

49 INVERTED TRIANGLE

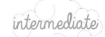

Parivrtha trikonasana

This pose improves the flexibility of your child's back and spine, and reinforces their arms, legs, and lower back. The twisting motion massages the intestines and improves digestion.

1. Stand up, legs wide apart. Extend your arms shoulder height, palms facing down. Inhale deeply.

2. Exhale as you twist your torso and hips to the right.

3. Position your left hand on the outside of your right foot, or as close to it as you can. Your right arm is aligned with your left arm and extended toward the ceiling. If at all possible, try to make sure you're looking at your left hand.

4. Come back to center and switch sides. Repeat three times, alternating sides.

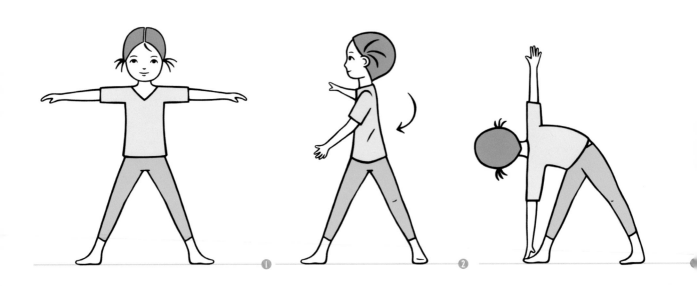

50 DIFFICULT *Ugrasana*

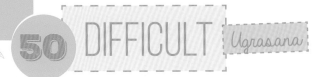

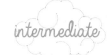

This pose strengthens your child's legs and stimulates their digestive organs. It improves the irrigation and oxygenation of the brain.

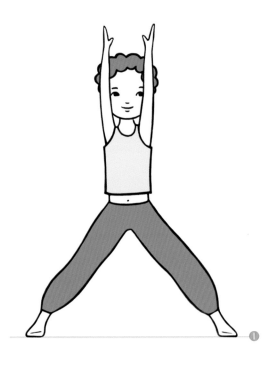

1. Stand up, legs apart as much as you can. Extend both arms above your head.

2. Bend forward and put your hands (or fingers, if easier for you) on the floor.

3. Touch the floor with the top of your head (opening your feet will help). Try touching your toes with your hands. Remain in position for a few moments, breathing normally.

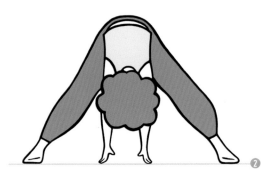

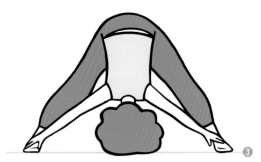

51 STAFF *Dhandasana*

This pose stretches your child's spine as well as their calves and back muscles.

1. Sit with your legs extended in front of you, your feet together, and your toes pointing to the ceiling.

2. Put your hands flat on the floor, giving a light push.

3. Inhale and exhale deeply several times.

4. You can practice the pose with your eyes shut or open.

Practice with your child. Just like the standing postures, the sitting postures (activities 51 to 66) usually become more appealing when practiced as a game. For example, while in upward plank you can let a ball roll down the child's back.

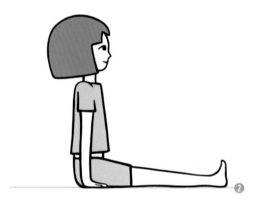

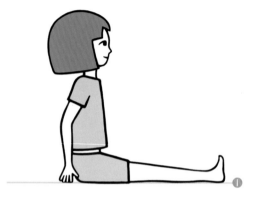

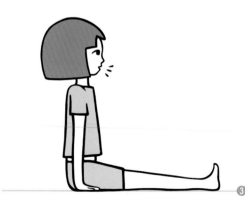

52 UPWARD PLANK (TOBOGGAN) *Purvottanasana*

This posture strengthens the arms and wrists of your child. It also improves the range of their shoulder movements and stretches the torso.

1. Sit with your legs extended in front of you, your feet together, and your toes pointing up.

2. Place your hands flat on the floor by your hips, fingers pointing in front of you.

3. Slightly bend your knees so your feet are flat on the floor.

4. While inhaling, bring your body up, keeping your arms and legs extended. The whole body is stretched, head back, and torso arched. Hold the pose for a whole breathing cycle.

5. Exhale while going back to your initial position.

6. Repeat three times.

> *You can help your child lift up their body so the stretch is easier.*

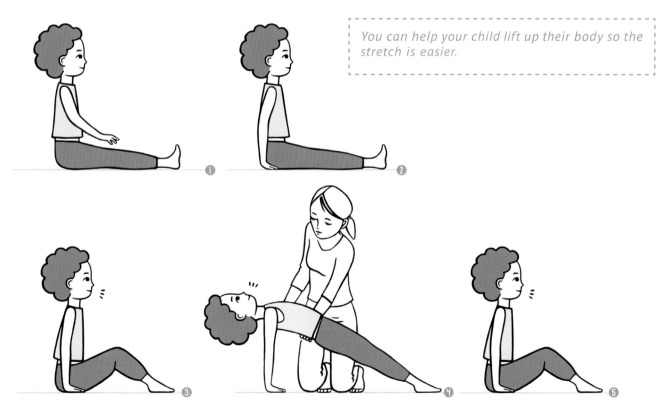

53 HEAD-TO-KNEE FORWARD BEND

Janu sirsasana

beginner

This pose stretches your child's spine and shoulders. It is recommended to dissipate headaches, stimulate the liver and kidneys, and facilitate digestion.

1. Sit with your legs extended in front of you.

2. While breathing, bring your right foot to your pelvis, sole touching your left thigh.

3. Turn your torso to the left.

4. While exhaling, bend forward and grab the foot or the ankle of the extended leg. Breathe normally for a few seconds.

5. Switch sides.

6. Repeat two or three times, alternating sides.

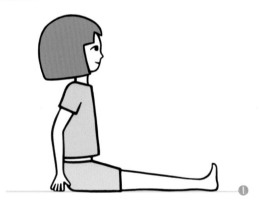

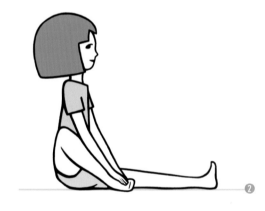

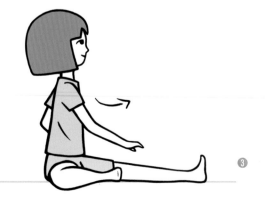

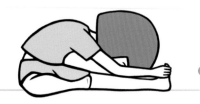

54 SEATED-FORWARD BEND

advanced

Paschimottanasana

This pose improves blood circulation, irrigating the muscles of the back by stretching them from the nape to the heels, including the back of the thigh muscles. It also calms the mind and helps to alleviate your child's stress.

1. Sit with your legs extended in front of you.

2. Keep your feet together, with your toes pointing up toward the ceiling.

3. Breathe in while bringing your arms up.

4. Exhale as you bend forward and grab your big toe.

5. Without straining too much, try to touch your knees with your forehead.

6. Hold the pose and count to three.

7. Inhale as you come back up, arms toward the ceiling.

8. Exhale and bring both of your arms down by your hips.

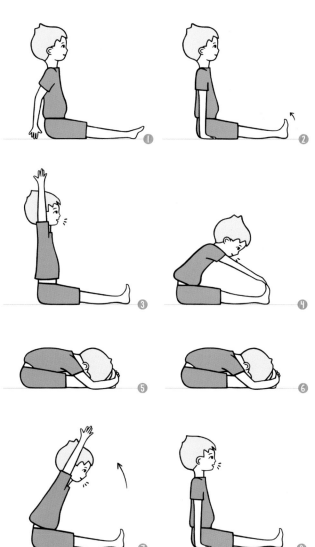

55 WIDE-ANGLE SEATED-FORWARD BEND

Upavistha konasana

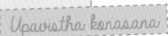

This pose improves your child's lower back, thigh, and calf flexibility. It also expands their hip and shoulder range.

1. Sit with your legs extended in front of you.

2. Open your legs wide, keeping your knees straight.

3. Inhale while bringing your arms up.

4. Exhale while bending down. Grab your big toes with your hands.

5. Flexible children can touch the floor with their forehead.

6. Hold the pose and count to three.

7. Inhale as you come back into the initial position.

8. Repeat three times.

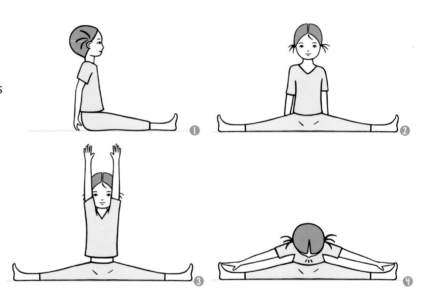

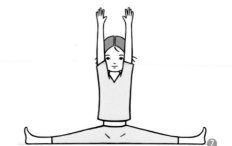

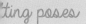

56 TORTOISE Kurmasan

This pose improves the child's lower back flexibility. It expands their hip and shoulder range, making forward stretching easier. It tones the back, thigh, and hip muscles.

1. Sit with your legs extended in front of you and engaged.

2. Open your legs as much as you can, then bend them slightly.

3. Weave your arms under your knees, palms towards the floor.

4. Bend forward and try to touch the floor with your chin. Push your heels upward to bend your torso with more ease.

5. Hold the pose for a few seconds, breathing normally.

6. Slowly come back to the initial position.

7. Repeat three times.

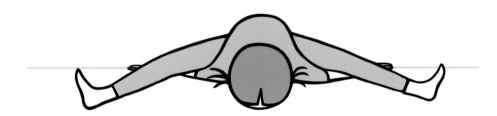

57 ARCHER 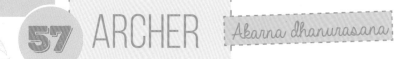 *Akarna dhanurasana*

The nerve of the big toe is linked to that of the abdomen, so there are many benefits to the abdomen when practicing this pose. It improves hip flexibility, strengthens the arms, and develops the child's balance.

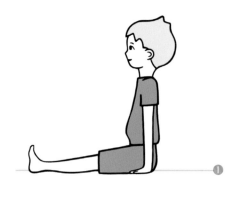

1. Sit with your legs extended in front of you.

2. Bend your left leg by bringing your left knee to your torso.

3. Grab your left big toe with your left hand and pull your leg up, bringing your foot close to your left ear.

4. If at all possible, grab your right big toe with your right hand. Try to hold the pose while breathing normally.

5. Switch sides.

If it helps, your child can use both hands to bring their foot up to their ear.

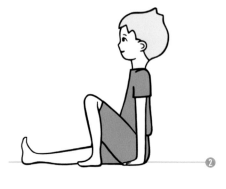

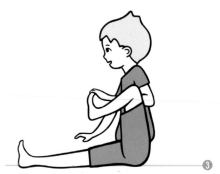

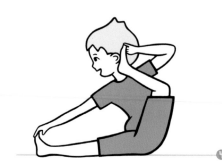

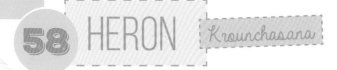

58 HERON *Krounchasana*

This pose stretches the back of the child's leg muscles. It also stimulates the abdominal organs and the heart.

1. Sit with your legs extended in front of you.

2. Fold your right leg under your right hip.

3. Using both hands, grab your left foot.

4. Progressively raise your left leg, keeping it extended at all times.

5. Try touching your leg with your forehead (if possible). Hold the pose a few seconds, breathing normally.

6. Switch sides.

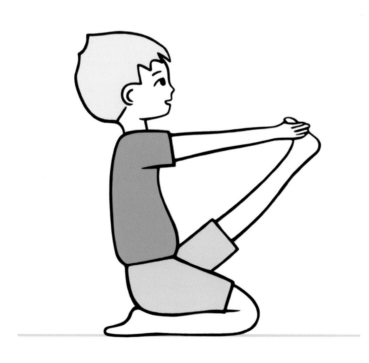

59 BOAT *Navasana*

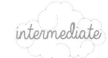

This pose reinforces back, abdominal, and hip flexors. It also improves your child's balance and concentration.

1. Sit with your legs extended in front of you, feet together.

2. Bend your knees, bringing them to your torso.

3. Extend your arms forward by your knees.

4. Slightly tilt your torso backwards.

5. Extend your legs, toes pointing upward.

6. Stay in this V-shape for a few seconds, breathing normally.

7. Bend your knees, feet on the floor.

8. Come back to the initial position, legs extended in front of you.

9. Repeat three times.

You can help your child hold the pose.

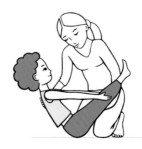

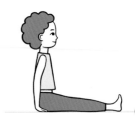

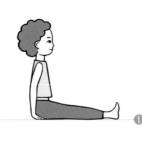

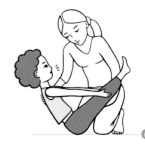

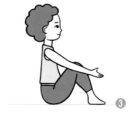

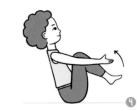

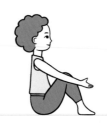

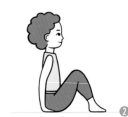

60 BOUND ANGLE (BUTTERFLY)

Baddha konasana

This pose stretches the child's spine, backs of the thighs, groin, and knee muscles. It also improves the flexibility of the ligaments and of the muscles in the pelvis area.

1. Sit with your legs extended in front of you, feet together.

2. Bring both feet as close to you as you can, soles anchored on the floor.

3. Keeping your feet together, open your legs as much as you can. Join your hands and place them around your toes. Keep your spine straight.

4. Hold the pose as long as you can while breathing deeply several times. Repeat three times.

5. Dynamic variation: after you have held the pose long enough, move your legs up and down like the wings of a butterfly.

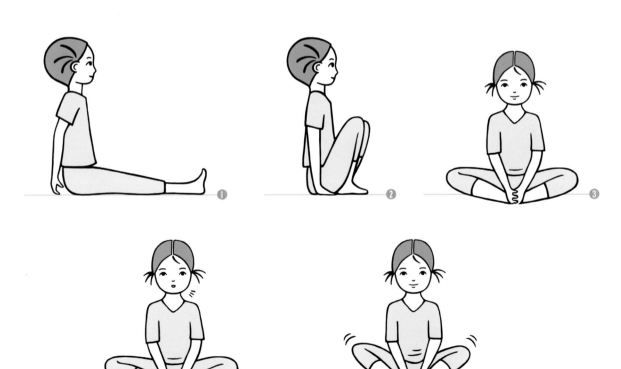

71

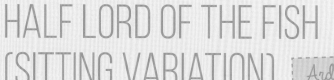

61 HALF LORD OF THE FISH (SITTING VARIATION)

Ardha matsyendrasana

advanced

This pose stretches your child's back muscles and improves the flexibility of the spine. It also stimulates the stomach, intestines, kidneys, and facilitates digestion.

1. Sit with your legs extended in front of you.

2. Bend your right leg, bringing the right foot to the outside of your left knee.

3. Fold the left leg, bringing your left foot to the right of your right hip.

4. Twist your torso to the right as much as possible.

5. With your left hand, grab your right ankle. Your left elbow is on the exterior of your right knee,

supporting your weight in the front. Your extended right arm, parallel to your body, supports your weight in the back.

6. Switch sides, inverting the crossing of your legs and twisting your torso to the left.

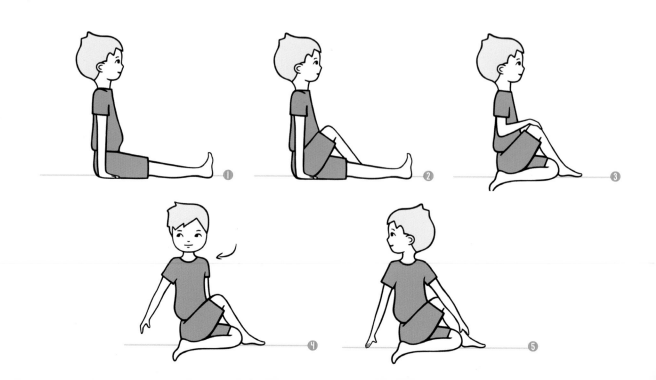

62 COW FACE *Gonukhasana*

This pose provides relief and flexibility to your child's shoulders. It tones the back muscles and helps align the spine. It also prevents sciatica pain.

1. This pose can be practiced sitting or standing. As a sitting posture, sit with your legs extended in front of you.

2. Bend your right leg to bring your foot back over the inside of your left knee.

3. Bend your left leg and bring your foot next to your right hip.

4. Try to bring the right foot as close to your left hip as possible.

5. Sitting or standing, bring your right arm up and bend it behind your back as you inhale. Bend your left arm behind your back and grab your right hand. Breathe normally for at least three seconds.

6. Come back to the original position. Switch sides. Depending on the child, this pose might be easier on one side.

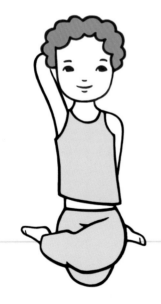

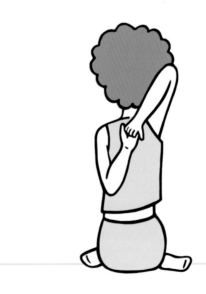

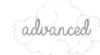

63 CAMEL *Ustrasana*

This pose tones and increases the flexibility of your child's spine, hips, and thighs. It improves shoulder range, while stretching the torso and the abdominal organs.

1. Start in a kneeling position.

2. Push your hips forward and slightly arch your back.

3. Place your hands on your ankles.

4. Very progressively arch your back.

5. Hold the pose, counting to three and breathing deeply.

6. To get out of pose, push your body forward as you let go of your ankles one after the other.

7. Repeat three times.

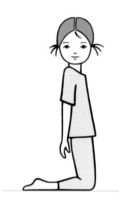

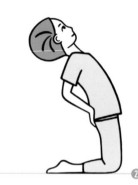

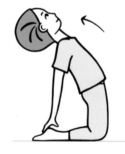

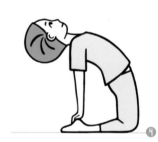

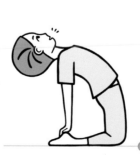

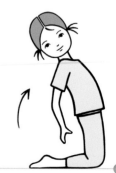

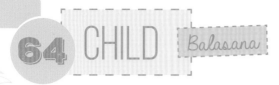 **64 CHILD** Balasana

This pose increases the flexibility of your child's back, leg, and ankle muscles. It also provides a total relaxation.

1. Start in a kneeling position and sit on your heels.
2. Bend forward and rest your forehead on the floor.
3. Keep your arms back along your body.
4. Repeat three times.

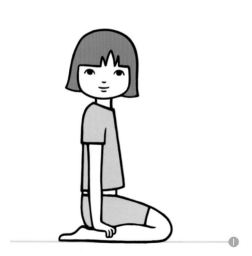

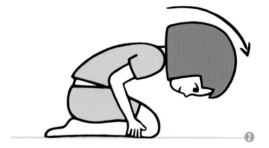

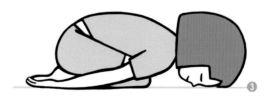

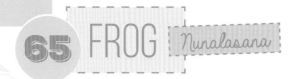

65 FROG *Nunalasana*

This pose stretches the back muscles and improves spine flexibility.

1. Sit on your heels.

2. Bend forward, placing your forearms and hands flat on the floor.

3. Tilt your head up and look right in front of you, like a frog. Hold the pose a few seconds, breathing normally.

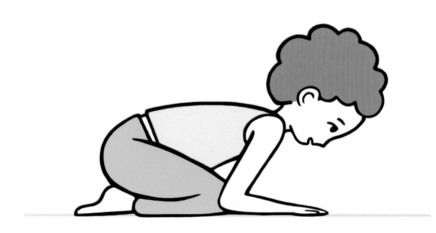

66 ONE-LEGGED KING PIGEON

Ekapada raja kapotasana

This pose stretches the child's thighs, abdomen, torso, and neck. It opens the hips as the legs are splayed. It also opens the thorax and improves lung capacity.

1. Start on all fours.

2. Bend the right leg to bring your right foot by your left thigh.

3. Slide the left foot back, extending your leg fully. Your right foot is half way between your left hand and thigh.

4. Bringing your hands closer to your body, find your balance so your back and face are upright. Hold the position while taking three normal breath cycles.

5. Switch sides.

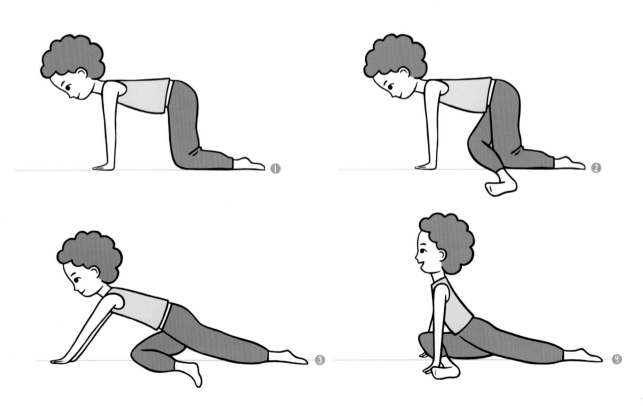

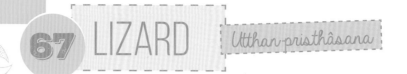

67 LIZARD

Utthan-pristhâsana

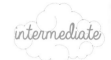

This pose tones the thighs, legs, and hips. It opens your child's torso and hips. Additionally, it improves the flexibility of the knees, wrists, and elbows.

1. Start on all fours.

2. Bring your left foot flat to the outside of your left hand.

3. Extend the right leg backward.

4. Bend your elbows and place your forearms on the floor.

5. Lower your stomach as close to the floor as you can. You are a lizard basking in the sun. Hold the pose for a few seconds, breathing normally.

6. Switch sides.

> *Like the standing or sitting postures, the lying postures (activities 67 to 83) can be realized in sequences, with forward-backward stretching, spine twisting, and open leg variations. Their objective is essentially to improve spine flexibility and body relaxation (crocodile, happy baby). It is recommended that the poses be practiced on a mat or a firm and flat floor, but not on a bed.*

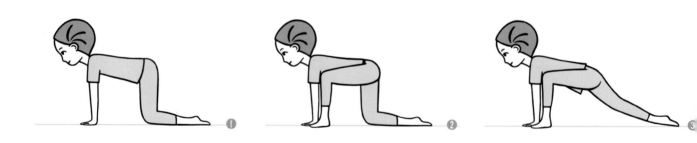

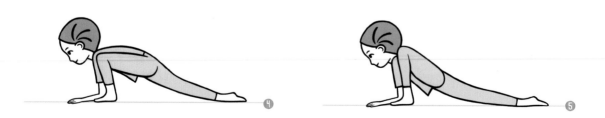

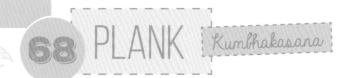

68 PLANK *Kumbhakasana*

This pose tones your child's spine. It also strengthens their shoulders, arms, wrists, abdominals, buttocks, and thighs.

1. Lie on your stomach.

2. Bring your hands flat at shoulder level and curl your toes for extra support.

3. and 4. Pushing on your arms up, raise your upper body. The arms are extended, so the body forms a straight line, like a plank.

5. Breathe normally and hold the pose for five to ten seconds.

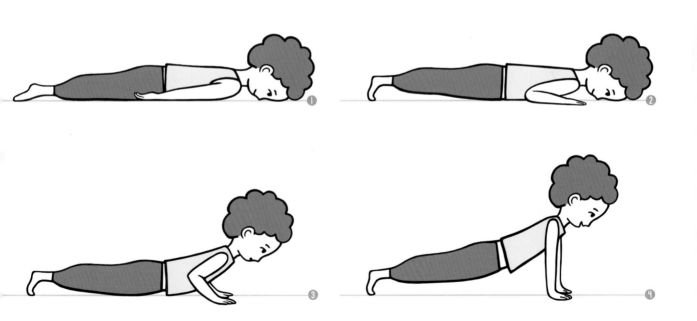

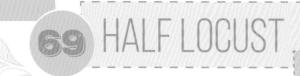

69 HALF LOCUST

Ardha salabhasana

This pose allows the child to feel their back. As it strengthens it, it stimulates the abdominal organs. It also reinforces the neck, leg, and thigh muscles while toning the arms, glutes, and legs.

1. Lie on your stomach, arms along your body, forehead on the floor.

2. Slightly raise your head to bring your chin onto the floor, and gaze ahead.

3. While inhaling, raise your foot up, extending your leg without bending your knee or ankle. The rest of your body remains flat on the floor.

4. Try to hold the pose a few seconds while breathing normally.

5. As you exhale, bring your foot back down.

6. Switch sides.

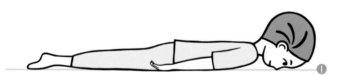

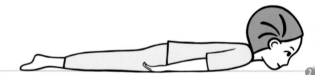

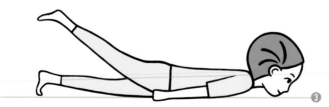

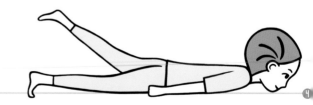

70 LOCUST *Salabhasana*

This pose strengthens your child's lower back, stomach, thighs, arms, and neck.

1. Lie on your stomach.

2. Arms are along your body, palms facing up.

3. and 4. Breathe while raising your legs, your torso, and your arms. Raise your head and look in front of you, if possible.

5. Slowly bring your feet, your torso, and your arms back down as you exhale.

6. Repeat three times.

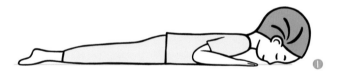

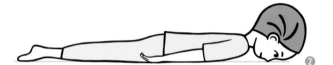

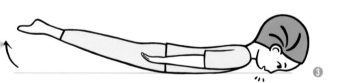

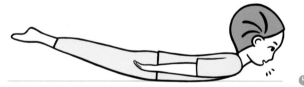

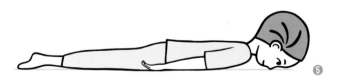

71 INVERTED BOAT

Viparita navasana

This pose improves your child's hip and spine flexibility by relaxing them. It strengthens the muscles of the back, and opens the torso, diaphragm, and solar plexus. Because the pose promotes breathing, it is recommended for stressed, tense, and nervous children.

1. Lie on your stomach, with your forehead on the floor.

2. Extend your arms above your head.

3. While inhaling, raise your arms and legs. Stop breathing and keep your balance as you hold the pose.

4. Exhale while coming back to your initial position.

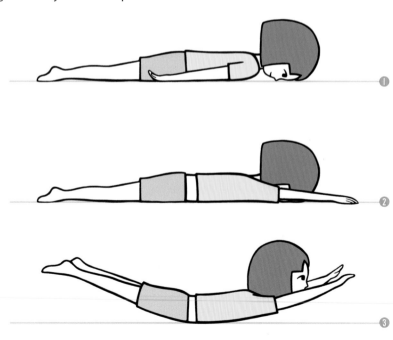

72 COBRA *Bhujangasana*

**This pose strengthens your child's spine and glutes.
It also works the torso, lungs, shoulders, and abdomen.**

1. Lie on your stomach and put your legs together.

2. Bring your hands to shoulder level, keeping your forehead on the floor.

3. and 4. While inhaling, raise your torso and look up to the sky.

5. and 6. While exhaling, come back to the initial position, forehead on the floor.

7. Repeat three times.

Your child can look straight ahead, arms slightly bent, or look up, arms extended. You can ask the younger ones to hiss like a cobra.

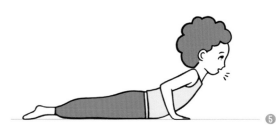

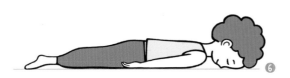

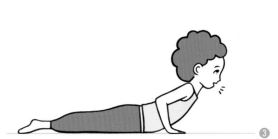

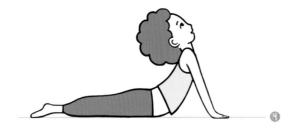

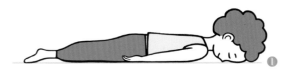

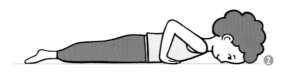

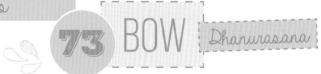

73 BOW *Dhanurasana*

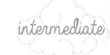

This pose strengthens the muscles of your child's back, stomach, thighs, arms, and neck. It increases spine flexibility and hip and shoulder mobility. It also massages the abdominal organs.

1. Lie on your stomach, with your feet extended and your arms at your side.

2. Inhale while bending your legs to bring your heels on your buttocks.

3. Grab your ankles with your hands.

4. Lift your head, upper body, and thighs, then look right in front of you.

5. Your body has the shape of a bow.

6. Exhale while coming back to the original position.

7. Repeat three times.

You can help your child hold the pose.

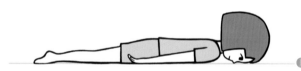

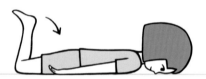

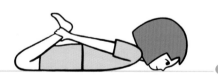

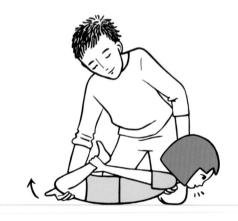

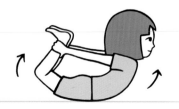

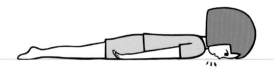

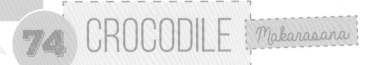

74 CROCODILE *Makarasana*

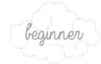

This pose is beneficial to the spine, and therefore to the nervous system. It stretches the back muscles and the glutes. It will help your child relax and fall asleep.

1. Lie on your stomach, forehead on the floor.

2. Raise your head, bend both of your arms, and bring your hands together to form a V-shape in which you rest your chin. Extend your legs, soles facing upward.

3. Slightly open your legs. Turn your feet inward so your heels touch the floor. Cross your arms to rest your forehead. Breathe normally for a few moments.

4. Bring your legs together and slowly get back up.

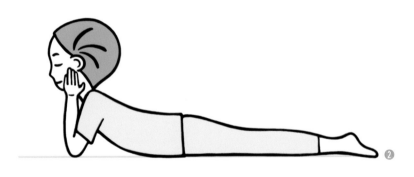

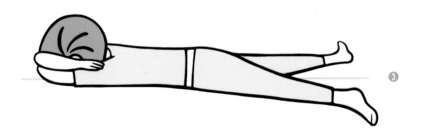

75 SLEEPING VISHNU (SIDE-RECLINING LEG LIFT)

Ananthasana

beginner

This pose improves leg flexibility and blood circulation. It is beneficial for your child, particularly for the heart and the digestive process.

1. Lie on your back and turn on your left side.

2. Bend your left arm so that you can rest your head on your left hand.

3. Bend the right leg and grab your right foot's big toe.

4. While inhaling, extend your leg up. Breathe in and out three times.

5. Bring your foot back on the floor while exhaling.

6. Switch sides

This posture can be practiced against a wall for better balance. If your child has difficulty reaching their big toe, tell them to reach their ankle or calf.

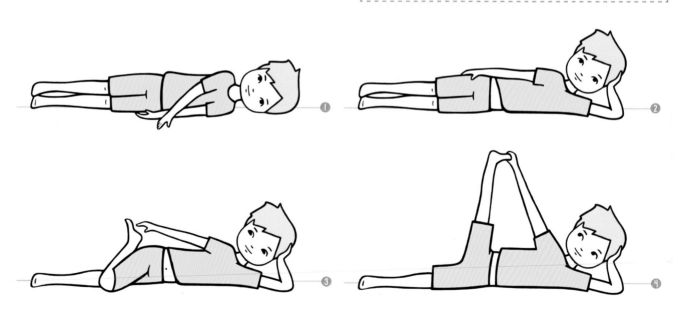

76 INVERTED LORD OF THE FISH (TORSION)

Supta matsyendrasana

This pose stretches the back muscles and glutes of your child. It relaxes the hips and back joints, and also stretches and realigns the spine. The twist massages the intestines and improves the digestive process.

1. Lie on your back, arms extended perpendicularly to your body.

2. Legs extended, twist your hips to the left, bringing your right foot close to your left hand, so you can grab your big toe.

3. Slowly turn your head to the right. Breathe deeply for a few seconds.

4. Come back to your initial position and switch sides.

If the big toe is too difficult to reach, the knee can slightly be bent.

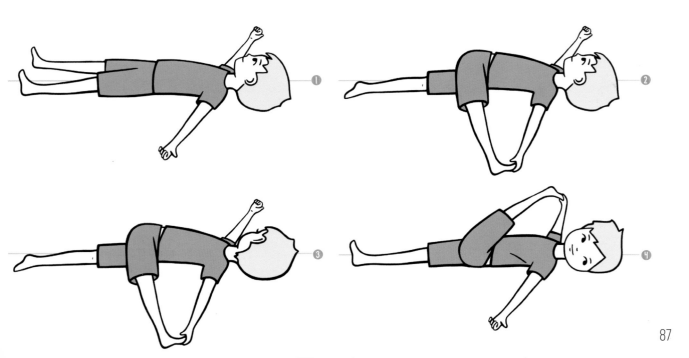

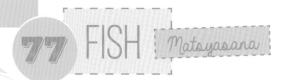 **77 FISH** *Matsyasana*

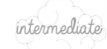

This pose improves your child's spine flexibility and strengthens the lower back, neck, shoulders, and arms.

1. Lie on your back, legs extended, arms along your body.

2. to 4. While inhaling, lift your torso, bring your shoulder blades together and gently place the back of your head on the floor. Use your elbows and forearms for support.

5. Slowly come back to the lying position while exhaling. Repeat three times.

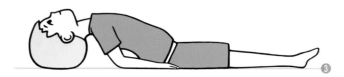

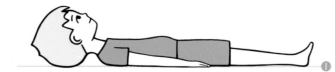

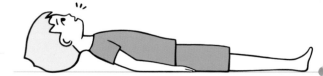

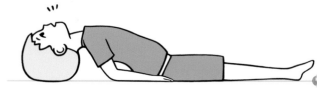

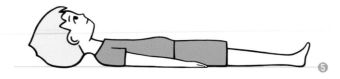

78 BRIDGE

Setu bandha sarvangasana

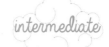

intermediate

This pose strengthens your child's lower back muscles and improves their spine flexibility. It also opens the torso, improves blood flow to the brain, stretches the neck and back, and helps the digestive system by stimulating the abdominal organs, the lungs, and the thyroid.

1. Lie on your back with your legs bent and knees up.

2. Grab your ankles with your hands. Inhale while lifting your buttocks as high as possible to form a bridge. Curve your lower back, bringing your torso close to your chin.

3. Try to let go of your ankles, placing your hands flat on the floor, or joining them under your back. Try to hold the position for a few seconds, breathing normally.

4. As you exhale, come back to the original position.

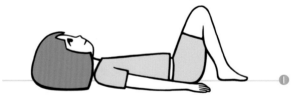

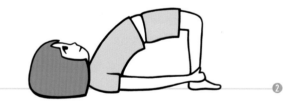

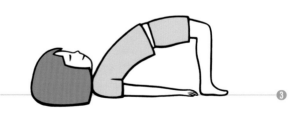

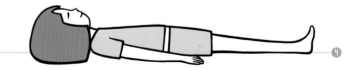

79 RECLINING HERO *Supta virasana*

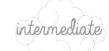
intermediate

This relaxation pose improves the flexibility of the abdomen, thighs, knees, ankles, and lumbar area. It also improves digestion and helps your child manage their stress by relieving tension.

1. Sit on your heels with your legs bent and back straight.

2. Open your legs and place your feet on each side of your thighs, bringing your buttocks to the floor.

3. Slowly place your elbows behind you and lie down progressively.

4. Your arms are extended on the floor above your head.

5. Try holding the position for a few seconds while breathing normally.

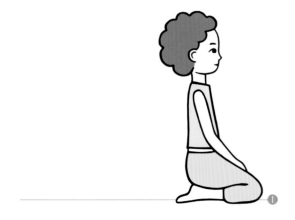

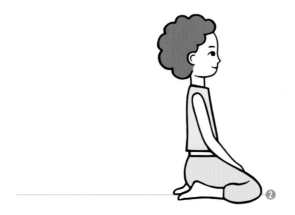

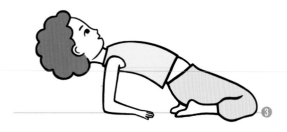

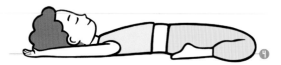

80 RECLINING BOUND ANGLE

intermediate

Supta baddha konasana

This pose helps your child open their shoulders, groin, thighs, and hips so as to rest the spine. It also stimulates the digestive system and abdominal organs.

1. Sit with your back straight.

2. Bend your legs to bring your knees to your torso.

3. Slowly lie down, keeping your legs bent.

4. Bend your legs and bring your soles together, and open your knees like a butterfly opening its wings. Keep your arms relaxed along your body.

5. Keep the position for a minimum of three breathing cycles.

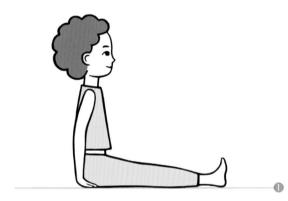

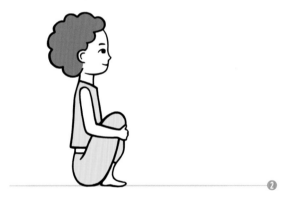

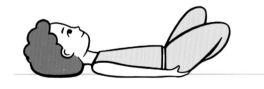

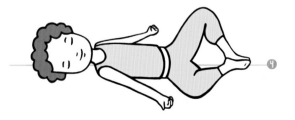

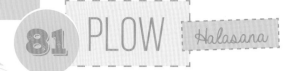

81 PLOW *Halasana*

This pose stretches your child's lower back. It promotes relaxation and mental calm, while improving digestion.

1. Sit with legs extended in front of you, feet together. Keep your arms along your body.

2. Tilt your torso backward, lifting your feet.

3. Continue tilting your feet backward so they end up touching the floor above your head.

4. Your arms remain on the floor, palms flat.

5. Stay in position for a few seconds, breathing normally.

6. Come back to the original position, legs bent.

7. Extend your legs.

8. Repeat three times.

For the more flexible:

9. Lying on the floor, tilt your body backward to bring your feet behind your head.

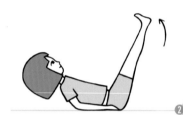

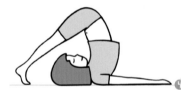

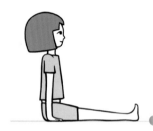

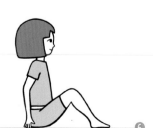

> *You can help your child hold the pose.*

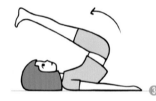

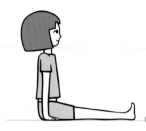

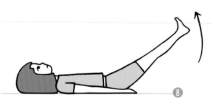

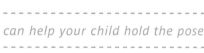

82 KNEE-TO-CHEST Apanasana

This pose stretches your child's lower back. It promotes relaxation and mental peace, while improving digestion.

1. Lie on your back.

2. Bend your knees and bring them to your chest while inhaling.

3. Put your arms around your knees. Hold the pose for a few seconds.

4. Go back to the original position while exhaling.

5. Repeat three times.

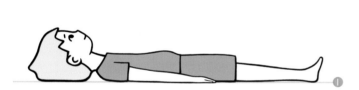

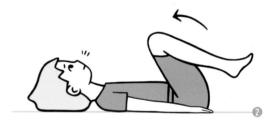

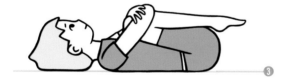

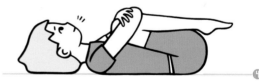

83 HAPPY BABY *Anandha balasana*

This pose improves the flexibility of your child's hips. It helps open shoulders, groin, thighs, and hips. It relaxes the spine, feet, legs, and arms.

1. Lie on your back, knees bent on your torso, feet to the ceiling.

2. Grab your big toes with your hands.

3. Keeping your feet pointed upward, open your legs while bringing your knees to the pits of your arms, like a happy baby.

4. Try to keep the position for a few seconds while breathing normally.

You can help your child be a happy baby.

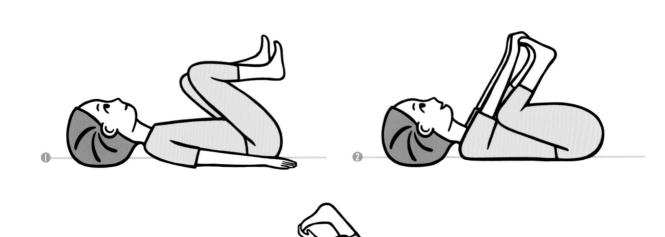

84 GARLAND *Malasana*

This pose improves the flexibility of your child's ankles. It stretches and tones the back and the lumbar area. It also tones the lower part of the legs and the neck muscles.

1. Stand, legs slightly apart.

2. Crouch down like a frog.

3. Join your hands in namaskar-mudra, or "salutation gesture," supporting your arms on the side of your knees.

4. Breathe normally for at least three seconds.

The "other postures" (activities 84 to 95) engage other elements of the body: eyes, face, brain, etc. They are mostly practiced head down, which enhances the blood flow to the brain. These positions are important. They should be practiced under an adult's supervision, and with scrupulous respect for the different steps. Although liked by children, wheel and pear tree are advanced poses. Face and eye yoga become yogic games when paired with voices and funny faces.

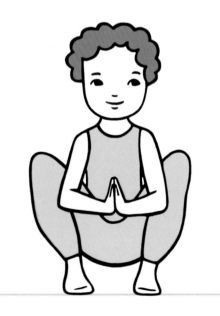

85 GATE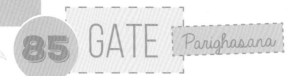

Parighasana

 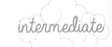
This pose improves the flexibility of your child's back, hips, spine, and thighs. It stimulates the abdominal organs and the lungs.

1. Kneel on a thick carpet or folded towel to protect your knees.

2. Extend your left leg on the side, keeping your heel on the floor. Anchor your right knee on the floor and curl your toes for extra support.

3. Slide your left hand onto your left leg so as to progressively reach your ankle, if possible.

4. Stretch your body to the left, right arm and fingers extended by your right ear, while looking up,

if possible. Hold the pose for a few seconds while breathing normally.

5. Come back to the initial position.

6. Switch sides.

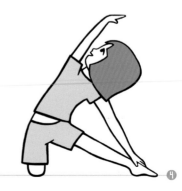

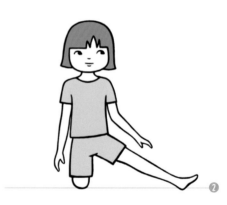

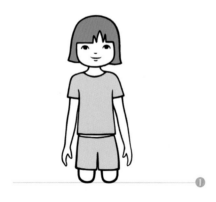

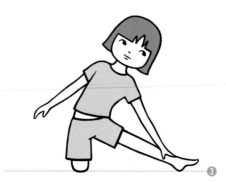

86 CAT AND COW *Marjaryasana*

This pose releases back and neck tensions. It also works the nape, arms, shoulders, digestive system, and eyes of your child.

Cat

1. Sit on your heels then get on all fours.

2. Round up your back, looking at your stomach while inhaling.

Cow

3. Assume the first step of Cat.

4. Push your back down, release your stomach muscles, and look up while exhaling.

5. Repeat three times, alternating poses.

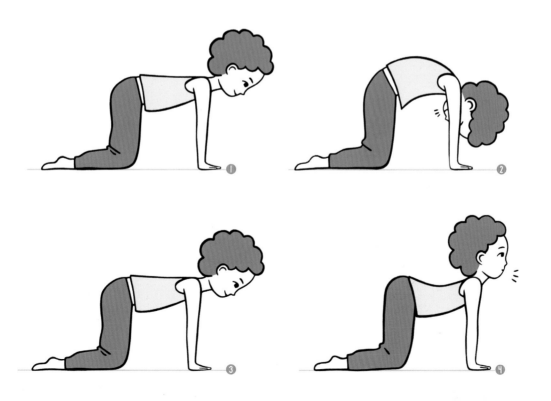

87 TIGER *Vyagarasana*
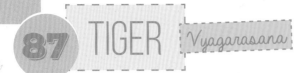

This pose stimulates your child's spine. It tones the legs, arms, shoulders, hips, and thighs. It improves balance and back muscle flexibility.

1. Get on all fours, hands aligned with your shoulders, knees aligned with your hips.

2. Breathe in as you bend and lift your right leg so your right foot is parallel to the floor (representing the tiger's tail).

3. Tilt your head back to look at the ceiling (or look ahead). Keep the arms on the floor for support. Hold the pose for at least three breathing cycles.

4. Switch sides.

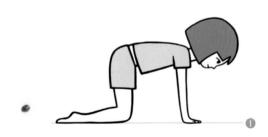

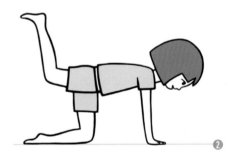

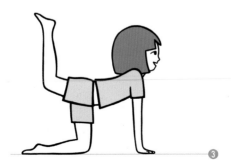

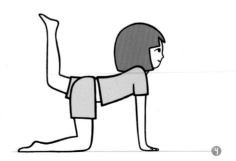

88 DOWNWARD-FACING DOG

beginner

Adhomukhasvanasana

This pose stretches your child's shoulders, calves, and hands. It strengthens arms and legs. If practiced with one leg up, it helps develop balance.

1. Get on all fours.

2. Put your weight on your hands. Inhale as you bring your buttocks up.

3. Legs and arms remain extended. Your head is in between your arms.

4. Try to lift one foot up and extend your leg, if possible.

5. Breathe normally, holding the pose for a few seconds.

6. Exhale as you come back to your initial position.

7. Repeat three times, alternating sides.

The younger ones might enjoy barking when in full pose. If the pose seems too difficult to do alone, help your child raise their leg up.

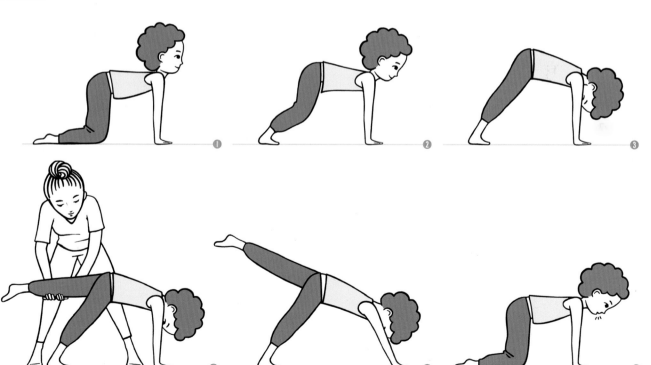

89 HALF-SUPPORTED HEADSTAND

intermediate

Ardha sirsasana

This pose tones thighs and heels. It promotes blood flow to the brain and eyes, contributing to the improvement of your child's memory. It also works on balance.

1. Place yourself against a wall. Kneel close to the wall and lower your torso to put your weight on your forearms, keeping your hands together.

2. Place your head on the floor, securely wedged between your hands.

3. Lift your buttocks toward the ceiling, keeping your legs extended.

4. Walk your feet toward you, so your back is straight against the wall. Look in the direction of your feet. Hold the pose for a few seconds, breathing normally.

You can offer a cushion or a folded towel to support your child's head.

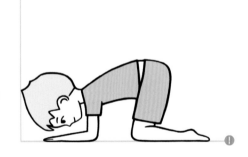

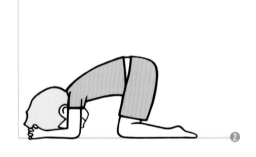

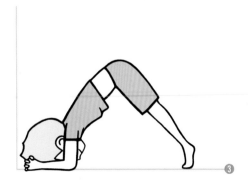

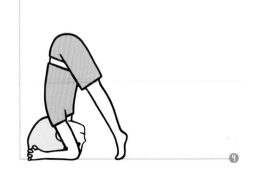

90 SUPPORTED HEADSTAND

Sirsasana

This pose is considered one of the best in yoga because it benefits the whole body. It improves the blood flow to the brain and eyes, and relieves a large number of muscles. It develops body balance and helps your child overcome the fear of being "head-down."

1. Place yourself in front of a wall. Kneel close to the wall; lower your torso to put your weight on your forearms.

2. Bend your arms so they are parallel to your thighs, your weight being supported by your hands.

3. Place the top of your head against the wall.

4. Lift your buttocks by extending your legs.

5. Lift one foot up.

6. Lift the other foot up. Your legs are both extended, feet together against the wall. Hold the pose for a few seconds while breathing normally.

7. Come back to the initial position by bringing one foot, then the other, back on the floor.

You can help your child by holding their first foot while their second leg goes up against the wall, then by making sure they are maintaining a good balance.

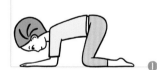

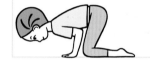

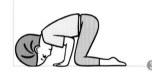

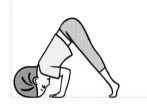

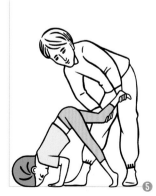

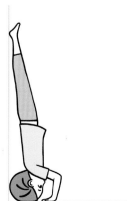

91 REVERSE TABLE TOP

Ardha purvottanasana

This pose improves the flexibility of your child's pelvis and joints. It strengthens the neck, arms, wrists, legs, shoulders, and abdomen. It opens the shoulders and chest.

1. Sit with your legs extended in front of you and slightly apart.

2. Place your hands on the floor by your hips, keeping your fingers pointing toward your feet.

3. Bend your knees toward your torso.

4. Inhale as you lift your stomach toward the ceiling to get into reverse tabletop. If possible, tilt your head back. Try to hold the pose for a few seconds, breathing normally.

5. Exhale as up bring your buttocks down to the floor. Rest for three breathing cycles.

As a yogic game, you can use your child's table-top by setting a light and stable object on it.

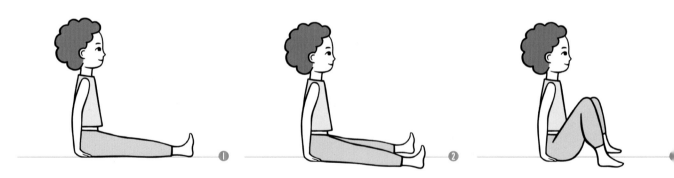

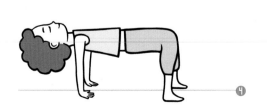

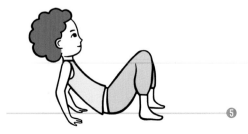

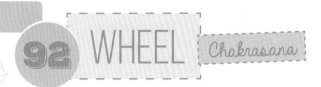

92 WHEEL *Chakrasana*

advanced

This pose improves the flexibility of your child's back and spine, while strengthening the arms, legs, and lower back.

1. Lie down on your back. Bend your knees, keeping your feet on the floor. Bring your heels to your buttocks and your arms above your head. Place the palms of your hands above your shoulders, with your fingers pointing toward your feet, elbows up.

2. Using your hands and feet for support, bring your body up. If possible, your head is lifted off the floor.

Children usually like wheel. For the first few times, adults can help the child raise and lower their hips. For the youngest, the top of the head can stay in contact with the floor.

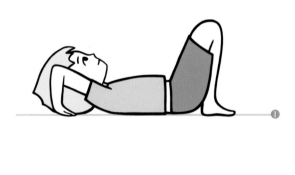

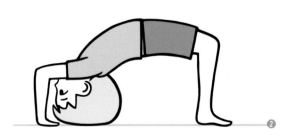

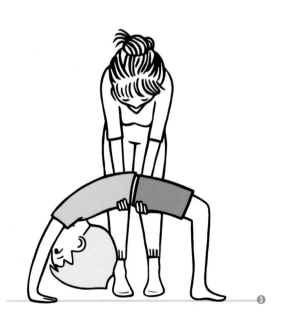

other poses

93 EYE YOGA 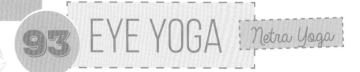 *Netra Yoga*

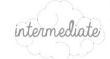

intermediate

These facial movements stimulate and strengthen your child's eye muscles. The eye is relaxed and irrigated, improving its performance. These exercises also relieve tired eyes.

1. Sit comfortably keeping your back straight.

2. Look up, then in front of you.

3. Look down, then in front of you.

4. Look right, then in front of you.

5. Look left, then in front of you.

6. Look successively up right, down left, up left and down right.

7. Slowly move your eyes in a circle, starting on one side.

8. Alternate sides at least five times.

Ask the child to hold each position for a few seconds. You can help orient their gaze with your finger or with an object.

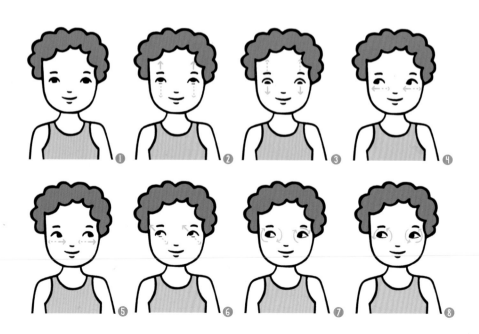

94 FACE YOGA · Mukha Yoga

These facial expressions stimulate your child's many facial muscles. They help tone the face and allow children to express their emotions and relieve their stress.

1. Sit comfortably with your back straight.

2. Puff up your cheeks as if they were balloons.

3. Let go of the air and pinch your inner cheeks with your teeth.

4. Make a big smile by bringing your cheeks all the way to your ears.

5. Clench your teeth and open your lips to show all your teeth.

6. Pucker your lips as if sending a kiss, then lift your head as if kissing the sky.

7. Rotate your tongue in your mouth, between your teeth and the inside of your cheeks.

Ask your child to hold the expression for at least ten seconds. Between expressions, the child comes back to a neutral face, eyes closed and muscles relaxed.

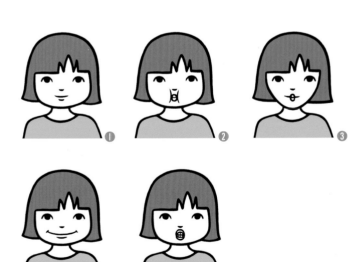

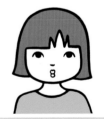

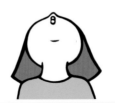

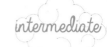

95 BRAIN YOGA *Thoppukaranam*

This pose, also called "super brain yoga," helps stimulate the brain. It is recommended that it be practiced every morning to improve concentration. Some schools make their pupils practice the pose at the beginning of the school day.

1. Stand up.

2. Bring your left hand to your right ear. Grab your right lobe with your left thumb on the side adjacent your face and your index finger behind the ear.

3. With your right hand, grab the lobe of your left ear with your thumb toward your face and index behind the ear. Stick your tongue against your palate.

4. Inhale, crouching down as far as you can without resting your buttocks on the floor.

5. Exhale, as you get back up.

6. Crouch down and come back up ten times without letting go of your lobes or moving your tongue from your palate.

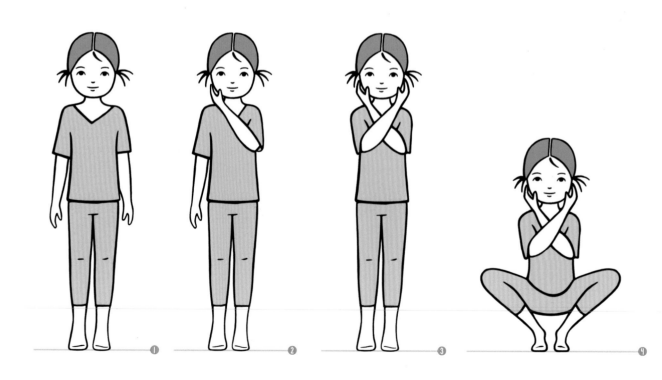

96 SCREAM Simhasana

This yogic game teaches children to inhale and exhale deeply. The angry lion prepares to roar on an inhale, and roars on an exhale. The exercise engages the muscle of the face, eyes, throat, and tongue.

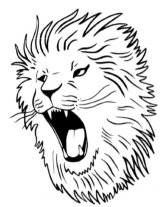

1. Kneel and sit on your heels.

2. Place the palms of your hands on your knees, keeping your fingers apart and extended.

3. Inhale, pushing out on your back and arching your shoulders.

4. Lower your head so you can see your belly button.

5. Exhale, sticking your tongue down and looking as far up as you can.

6. Scream like a roaring lion.

7. Stretch the muscles of your face to be as frightening as possible.

The yogic games (activities 96 to 100) aim to improve balance and concentration. They help your child perceive the many capabilities their body offers while motivating them to practice yoga. The sound games allow the child to exteriorize and relieve stress. They can be practiced anywhere, anytime, individually, or in a group.

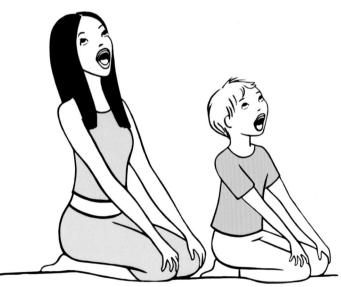

97 BREATH

This yogic game teaches children to master their breath, keeping it long and sustained.

1. Kneel and sit on your heels. Place a crumpled paper tissue in front of you. Softly blow on it to push it forward.

2. Lie on your back. Place a paper tissue on your mouth. Breathe out so as to see the tissue float as high as possible above your face.

To make the game more challenging, give your child limits or objectives, and replace several short breaths by a few long ones. You can also propose a contest.

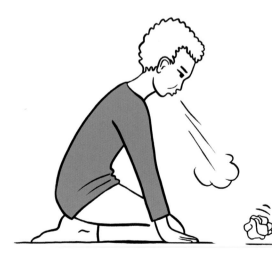

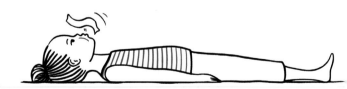

98 SOUND

This yogic game stimulates your child's face, throat, and respiratory system.

1. Sit comfortably in one of the four following yoga postures: easy (p.18), diamond (p.19), half-lotus (p.17), or lotus (p.17).

2. Breathe deeply, then exhale very slowly, making a very soft, continuous sound suitable for a relaxing meditation. You can choose one of the following: "Eeeeeeeeeeeeee", "Mmmmmmmmmmmm", "Ooooooooooooooo", "Aaaaaaaaaaaaa, (mouth wide open for the A sound).

Depending on the chosen sound, the child will exhale through the mouth or nose. This game can also be a contest, counting the seconds to determine each of the participants' endurance.

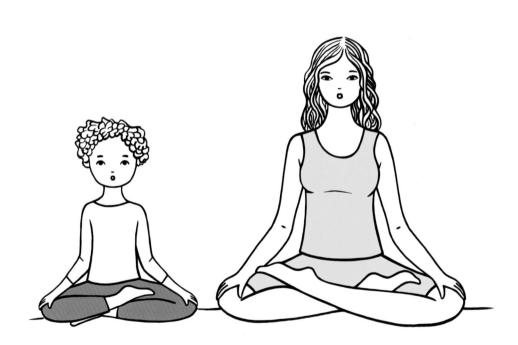

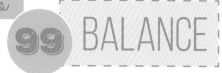

99 BALANCE

This yogic game improves balance and concentration. It strengthens the leg muscles. This game is very much liked by children who want to prove they can hold the pose for a long time.

1. Take one of the following yoga poses: Lord of the dance (p. 45), tree (p. 46), warrior III (p. 47), kite (p. 48), or any other pose on one foot.

2. Standing on one foot, try to hold the pose as long as possible.

This game can be turned into a timed competition between children, or between adult and child.

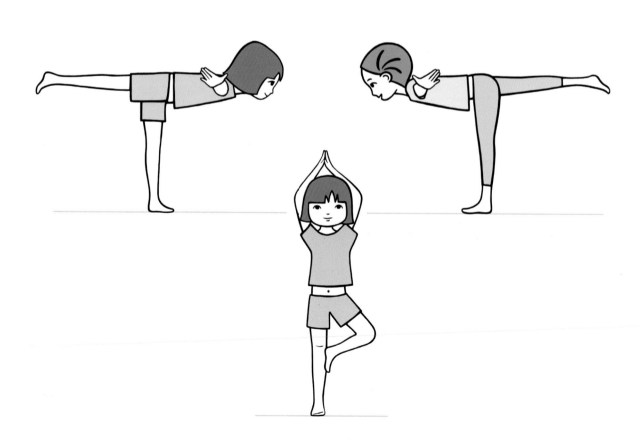

100 CONCENTRATION AND REFLEXES

This yogic game improves your child's concentration and reflexes while playing. It also improves the memorization of the poses.

1. This game starts from any simple posture (standing, sitting, or lying). You can add two similar poses, for example: crocodile (p. 85) and cobra (p.83); cat (p. 97) and dog (p. 99); crocodile (p. 85) and inverted boat (p. 82); locust (p. 81) and cobra (p. 83).

2. To work on concentration, repeat the same pose twice in a row: cobra, dog, cobra, dog, cobra, dog, cobra, dog, cobra, dog, dog, cobra, cobra. . . . Or, for the younger children, repeat the arms, legs, and eye movements on one side and then the other.

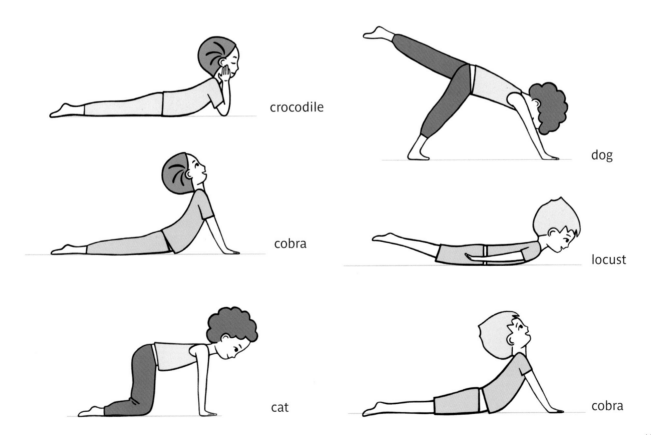

crocodile

dog

cobra

locust

cat

cobra

First United States printing 2017 by Skyhorse Publishing

Skyhorse Publishing books may be purchased in bulk at special discounts for sales promotion,
corporate gifts, fund-raising, or educational purposes. Special editions can also be created to
specifications. For details, contact the Special Sales Department, Skyhorse Publishing, 307
West 36th Street, 11th Floor, New York, NY 10018 or info@skyhorsepublishing.com.

Skyhorse® and Skyhorse Publishing® are registered trademarks of Skyhorse
Publishing, Inc.®, a Delaware corporation.

Visit our website at www.skyhorsepublishing.com.

10 9 8 7 6 5 4 3 2

Translation by François Gramet

Interior photography © iStockphoto
Illustrations by Oreli Gouel

Print ISBN: 978-1-5107-1959-0
Ebook ISBN: 978-1-5107-1960-6
Previous ISBN: 978-2-317-01749-0

Printed in China